TAKING CONTROL OF FIBROMYALGIA

FOLLOWING SCIENCE ON A NATURAL PATH TO HEALTH

CAROLINE WILLIAMS

TRISTARR PUBLISHING

INTRODUCTION

LOSING YOUR LIFE TO PAIN – AND GETTING IT BACK AGAIN

Tell me if this sounds familiar:

You've spent another restless night staring at the ceiling, shifting from side to side, trying to get comfortable. You hurt everywhere. There are all kinds of pains – stabbing pains, aching pains, pains that jump around like shocks of electricity. Your skin feels tight. Your head feels like it's full of cement. Dragging yourself out of bed to start another day feels like an insurmountable task. And when people ask what's wrong, you don't know how to explain it to them because you *look* fine.

You don't have any broken bones. You don't have a nasty rash. You still smile and tell jokes. So, it can't be that bad, can it?

Except, it is.

But when you tell people that you have something called 'fibromyalgia', their eyes glaze over. Isn't that one of those chronic fatigue things? Something that's all in your head? Are you stressed? Maybe you just need to lie down for a few weeks?

Tell me if this sounds familiar too:

Deep down you still wonder if, somehow, it's your fault that you feel this way.

Well, I'm here to tell you *emphatically* that it's not. Fibromyalgia is real, and I'm going to help you finally understand what it is.

Taking back control

What you're about to read is not another 'how to manage your symptoms' fibromyalgia book. I'm sure you've waded through several of those already. I'm also sure that if the suggestions inside those books had worked, you wouldn't still be looking for answers.

Because, for many fibromyalgia sufferers, *answers* are what's missing from the narrative currently circulating in society.

Books. Doctors. Forums and support groups. They all have suggestions for how to manage the myriad symptoms that come along with a fibromyalgia diagnosis, but they don't seem to be able to tell you *why* you have fibromyalgia or what it is in any sufficient detail.

Fibromyalgia is often dismissed. When it isn't, it's described as a 'chronic pain condition' or a 'neurological pain condition'. But what those terms *mean* is left up to the patient to decide.

As someone who has always looked to science for answers, this does not sit easy with me.

As an acupuncturist, I have treated many stubborn, complex conditions that traditional medicine couldn't impact. But when increasing numbers of patients came to me for help managing their fibromyalgia, I was shocked to find that there was very little *real* information out there about this condition.

The usual methods that I would use to treat chronic pain didn't work well for fibromyalgia either. The drugs that patients were being prescribed didn't seem to work either. And no one seemed to be able to accurately describe what fibromyalgia was or why a person might develop it.

I'm pleased to say that this is *slowly* changing. The scientific community is paying more attention to fibromyalgia, and I have developed an acupuncture system that is getting very promising results.

For patients who are suffering *right now,* I believe that understanding your condition is the key to feeling well again.

If you don't understand what's happening in your body, how can you find the right treatments for you to begin healing?

If you don't understand why you're in pain, how can you start to *believe* that it's possible to come out of the fibromyalgia state and be *you* again?

If you don't understand that the way you feel is *not* your fault, how can you take back control?

Because you can take back control and you can be you again. There is a lot that you can do at home, without the need to hire a therapist, take drugs, or visit a life-coach, to help yourself recover. And by explaining exactly what's going on inside your body, and why you feel the way you do, I'm going to show you how.

How did writing this book come about?

My close friend Clair was diagnosed with fibromyalgia eleven years ago. She's a therapist, and she's not used to being told there's something she can't fix, so she set off on a 'trying-things' journey. Clair was determined to heal herself, but it took ten long, painful years to find the right combination of tools to help her feel better.

We have chronicled much of this journey in our co-authored book *From Fibromyalgia to Freedom*. However, instrumental in Clair's path back to wellness was the new acupuncture system that I designed to treat fibromyalgia.

During her very worst year, we finished developing a new Vagal Toning Acupressure System (VTA) for fibromyalgia, which proved to be helpful for her and many of my other patients. After seeing success with VTA, Clair was able to stop taking the pregabalin she had been using for two years. She had a couple of very difficult days coming off the last of the drugs and I was with her as she experienced hallucinations, anxiety, and paranoia. That week, I realised I couldn't just keep hoping that someone else would write a book about fibromyalgia. I realised that someone needed to shine a light on what this condition is and how it can be treated.

Clair is now pain free and has her fibromyalgia under control. She suffers occasional flare ups, but her life is unrecognisable compared to how it was a few years ago. She now understands her condition and knows exactly what to do to help herself when she begins to feel unwell. But there are too many people still suffering, people who could be helped with the kind of information that helped her.

My experience of treating chronic pain and fibromyalgia

I have been practising as an acupuncturist for over twenty years. In that time, I have resolved many kinds of chronic pain conditions that were not responsive to prescription medications, NHS physiotherapy, or surgery. Acupuncture has a good reputation for making changes to pain and I have always found this part of my practice extremely fulfilling.

Due to my success with treating various complex pain conditions, my attitude towards chronic pain is that it can often be changed or completely resolved. I am not alone; there are pain specialists all over the world saying that we can change pain, and that we need to understand it differently.

Earlier in my career, however, I found fibromyalgia extremely frustrating to treat. I struggled to make a change to the condition using the traditional treatment strategies I had studied. This didn't make sense to me. Acupuncture is so good at changing other kinds of pain, and seeing Clair struggle for years with fibromyalgia pushed me to look at the condition in more detail.

By understanding what was happening to create the symptoms, I was able to develop a new way to treat it. Using this system (which I will teach you in the tools section of the book) I have been able to get much better results for fibromyalgia clients.

Chronic pain is a problem for everyone

I strongly believe that we desperately need more information about how to change pain. Currently, across the world, one in twenty people have fibromyalgia and one in five people suffer from moderate to severe chronic pain. But too many of us are simply handed painkillers and told to accept our lot.

Today, many people in pain seem to receive the distinct impression – from doctors, mainly – that they could be responsible for causing their condition themselves. Hearing phrases that are used for chronic pain like 'learned pain' can make it feel like the condition is somehow under your control, or that you have done something to get yourself into this situation. I have listened to many people tell me that their doctor says the pain 'can't be there' and I have had a senior NHS physiotherapist tell me that 'depression causes pain', which is a complete misunderstanding of how pain and depression interact.

All of this makes it very difficult for people who are suffering from chronic pain conditions, like fibromyalgia, to find the right treatment and to manage the emotional side of living in pain.

But I can assure you that you are not responsible for creating a chronic pain state like fibromyalgia. And I hope that by sharing some of the science with you, you'll be able to take back control and start your journey to wellness.

As we progress through the book, I'm going to distill some of the complex information that's out there so that you can begin to understand your pain, why you have it, and what you can do to alleviate it.

Scientific papers are absolutely crammed full of acronyms and jargon, which can make finding the useful bits of information a slow and daunting process. Much of this information is written for other academics to read and contains detailed explorations of research processes. Sometimes, it feels a bit like disappearing down a rabbit hole to look for glimpses of wisdom. However, there is a lot of extremely useful information to be found, things that we can use in our ordinary lives, *if* we know where to look.

I'm going to take you on a short, guided tour around some current scientific knowledge, visiting theories that can help you in a practical way with fibromyalgia and putting them in terms you will understand. I'm also going to share the acupressure system that I developed and I hope that this combination of knowledge and practical tools will help you to resolve your pain – and many of the other symptoms that accompany it.

Losing your life to pain

Most doctors don't know why you have fibromyalgia, or how to get rid of it.

When diagnosed, it's easy to feel that you are completely on your own with an unpleasant and life changing internal experience. It's not clear how you might have got to where you are, and no-one offers clear advice about how to get out of it again. You are advised to learn to live with it. The drugs you are given don't really work. No-one can see your condition. And you find that you can't do all the things you used to do.

It can be pretty scary.

In my experience, there are too many doctors telling people that fibromyalgia is an 'incurable disease' and sending them home with drugs, when actually there is a lot of useful research with good information about fibromyalgia and chronic pain conditions.

'Incurable' only means that there isn't a drug or treatment solution that you can buy or swallow. It does not mean that you can't get well again!

What are the recommended strategies for chronic pain?

In the UK, NHS pain clinics teach strategies such as pacing yourself (not over-doing it), acceptance, mindfulness, and stress management, all of which are useful if your pain is going to be permanent.

Many chronic pain conditions are caused by ongoing physical damage, like in Rheumatoid Arthritis (where the immune system attacks the joints). However, fibromyalgia creates a particular kind of pain, and this type of pain can be changed.

Here is where I found the lack of information given to fibromyalgia clients to be especially poor; instead of outlining the differences in types of pain, fibromyalgia clients are treated as standard chronic pain clients and just given drugs. However, fibromyalgia pain isn't created by body damage, although it might have started from an injury or a surgery. Fibromyalgia pain occurs due to changes in brain programming and inflammation, and this is a kind of pain that we are able to change.

There is a lot of overlap between the different types of chronic pain, as we will be exploring shortly, but fibromyalgia is at the far end of the scale in the 'brain pain' category.

"If it hurts, why don't you just take a pill?"

Unfortunately, pain has few effective medicines to treat it. Over the last ten years, drug companies have scaled back on the development of new drugs for pain[1] because with so many body systems involved, pain is a very difficult condition to treat with drugs.

Opioid medicines have been the mainstay of pain relief, however the current 'opioid crisis' in the USA has demonstrated how dangerous and unhelpful these drugs can be when used for long periods of time.

Opioid drugs can actually make pain *worse* if they are used for long-term pain. Now, pain specialists are recommending that opioid drugs are only ever used for very short-term situations, like immediately after a surgery. Newer, modified opioids do exist, and they are working differently in the brains of rats, but human trials have not been done with these yet. So, currently there are no effective pills that can be given to people to treat chronic pain from fibromyalgia.

How can this book help me?

This book is about how to reverse the fibromyalgia state. By understanding the basics of the science you'll have a map of fibromyalgia and you'll be able to see how you got 'here'. Once you understand your own route to pain, you can plan your route out again.

Our knowledge about pain is changing, and with any new information it takes a while for everyone to hear it.

For instance, we used to think that pain was a kind of a signal that went from a part of the body that was damaged up a nerve to the brain. Now, we know that pain is an interpretation that the brain makes from the evidence it has. Those signals from a damaged body part are just warning signals and they can travel up multiple pathways to the brain, not just one nerve.

New self-help tools

Acupressure has long been used to help with pain and this book contains a set of new acupressure tools that I have developed specifically for fibromyalgia. [Acupressure is the application of a really tiny amount of pressure on the surface of the skin, directly over an acupuncture 'point'.] This new system builds on the research from bio-electric medicine and includes vagal nerve toning points, all of which I will explain later.

All of the self-help tools suggested in this book are affordable and can be done in your own home. Instead of wondering about 'trying things', this book intends to build some useful signposts for you in the foggy world of pain.

FINDING YOUR WAY

Who is this book for?

This is a book for people with fibromyalgia or 'centralised' pain, and for anyone who thinks they *might* have fibromyalgia. It could also be useful reading for people with other forms of chronic widespread pain. Essentially, it is for anyone who is interested in finding out why fibromyalgia or centralised pain occurs and what you can do to reverse it.

The diagnostic categories for fibromyalgia, chronic widespread pain (CWP), or centralised pain have become increasingly blurred as we understand more about these conditions. There are only slight differences between them and medical professionals now refer to them as a group. In this book I am going to use the term fibromyalgia to refer to them all.

Fibromyalgia is often diagnosed after someone has been suffering for many years. The symptoms can develop slowly but addressing them early can be helpful.

When I started looking for information about fibromyalgia, I wanted to find out how it was caused and what we can do about it. I found lots of generalisations about how stress is 'linked' to fibromyalgia, and that the nervous system is involved, but with no real explanations about how this might connect with what a real person feels or does in their daily life.

To fill that gap, this book aims to be a straightforward guide to the biology behind the symptoms of fibromyalgia, so that you can use the information practically. Knowing this information could be the key to you getting rid of your pain as well as other symptoms you might be suffering with.

The key principles underpinning the chapters you're about to read are:

- Knowing how pain occurs is *useful.*
- Understanding that you can reverse the process is *essential.*
- Learning some tools that you can use *yourself,* and starting to get rid of your pain is *even better.*

Now, I know it's going to be tempting to skip ahead and look for the juicy bits; I do that myself. If an author promises us solutions, we often feel we'd like a quick bullet point version that will allow us to start implementing change.

But I *urge* you not to do that with this book.

This book, just like the self-help tools inside it, won't work if you just choose one area to focus on.

It is a bit like a recipe for one of those dishes that are in layers. A dish where you make the base, then the middle, and then the topping.

Each layer on its own is ok, but the dish is only amazing when it is all together and in the right order.

With this book, I will build a base for you with some simple biology about fibromyalgia, then the middle of our dish is to see how this relates to the other parts of us, and the topping will be the self-help tools, which will all make sense when the rest of the recipe is complete.

MAPPING THE TERRITORY

Where you might be now

There isn't a completely average fibromyalgia sufferer and you may have slightly different symptoms to another person, but it's likely that if you have full-blown fibromyalgia you are experiencing a combination of pain, fatigue, headaches, brain-fog, and maybe anxiety or depression with it.

Your pain could be a dull diffuse aching in muscles and joints, stabbing pains that wander about in the body, pins and needles, or a combination of all of these.

The fatigue you could feel can be mild or extreme, where dragging yourself out of bed every morning is a huge task. You may not feel like doing anything at all, but if you sit or lie down for too long the pains are worse.

It's likely that you have either been pushing through pain and tiredness or had to give up doing things you loved doing or were normal activities for you.

Headaches and neck pain are common, and they go along with a sense that the mind is foggy, your concentration is not as good as it was and its harder to stay focused and sharp.

The pain in fibromyalgia has an unusual quality. Fibromyalgia patients will often say they don't know if they can continue having this pain. It saps the joy out of life and feels unbearable. Other kinds of chronic pain don't have this unbearable quality. I believe it is because the pain feels all encompassing, without one specific location it has a sense of being everywhere.

There are over one hundred symptoms associated with fibromyalgia. We are going to start by looking at a basic map for this condition.

Landmarks on the way to fibromyalgia

The journey to get to a fibromyalgia state is slightly different for everyone, but it is likely that many of the same places are on most people's map.

1. At some point it is likely that you have experienced pain – an event like an accident, a surgery, or an injury that didn't seem to heal so well, or maybe an ongoing digestive problem.
2. It's also common that a stressful event or a period of intense stress may have occurred in your life.

We are going to explore these two types of events, pain and stress, to find out what might have happened to your body during and after them, because they show us how fibromyalgia can happen.

We'll start by looking at pain, looking at what the terminology means and at the kind of chronic pain that fibromyalgia creates.

What's different about chronic pain?

'Chronic' means something is ongoing, not temporary.

Most structural damage in the body is healed within about three months, so the question in medicine has always been 'What's going on when the patient says there is still pain after three months?'

Unfortunately, over the years some doctors have assumed that patients were just making it up or were super sensitive, and some doctors proposed that patients were converting repressed feelings into body pain and that therefore their pain was actually just a psychological problem.

This last explanation was especially dismissive because *everyone's* emotional feelings are felt in their body!

Fortunately, things have moved on and we know better now!

Responsibility for chronic pain conditions

Worldwide, we are in a transition process in the treatment of chronic pain. New information is out there but not everyone is aware of it yet. There is a considerable time lag in getting the new discoveries and thinking to everyone who needs to hear it.

Millions of people were hoping a doctor could fix their chronic pain or fibromyalgia for them, but people with these conditions are finding they have two options: either they accept that they are a 'broken human being' with some drugs to take, or they try to take control of the condition themselves.

The drugs we currently have aren't working very well on chronic pain, so even the first option isn't really practical, or comfortable.

In order to choose the second option, we need to educate ourselves about pain. I could warn you that this second option needs a little motivation, and the impetus to spend time on yourself to improve your health, but you already know that because you bought this book.

Different kinds of pain

One of the first things we can identify is whether a pain is *local* or *widespread.*

A typical kind of local pain is a muscle pain, which is called a myofascial pain. This is what most people experience as a normal muscle ache, caused by exercise, or from a damaged muscle like a sprain. Myofascial pain has only a *local* effect, meaning that the pain and fatigue effects are only felt in and around the muscles that are damaged.

In some people a local pain might be created by an ongoing structural issue - like arthritis, for instance, where there is damage to joints. If there is damage that can't be completely healed by the body it would show up as pain in specific areas around the damage, or running up or down from that place. (Local pain is also referred to as *peripheral* pain.)

In contrast, a widespread pain can affect any joint, muscle, or be in areas under the skin. This type of pain might be felt in the whole body. The pain can move about, appearing randomly in different places. The pain might come and go at different times of the day or night, and some days may be worse than others.

This is where the term '*centralised*' comes in. The pain is now coming from the central nervous system, rather than one specific (local) place. We will be exploring this idea as we go along to see what it means and what we can do about it.

Beware if you Google it that *centralised* pain is not the same as central pain syndrome!

Central pain syndrome is where there is actual damage to the spinal cord or brain, like in a stroke. *Centralised* pain (the one we are looking at) is a dysregulation in brain functioning which influences pain, but there is no damage to the brain or spinal cord.

Widespread and local pains tend to be treated differently.

- A local pain might be treated with exercise and physiotherapy or alternatively with surgery to repair or replace a part of the body.
- Widespread pain is more difficult to treat. Your doctor might give you anti-inflammatories or painkillers. These may help, allowing the body to heal, but alternatively the condition may not resolve and instead it becomes chronic. This is often the place that people find that the drugs stop helping or are creating unwanted side effects when taken long-term.

Pain can change!

The really important thing to know about these two categories of local or widespread pain is that a local pain can turn into a widespread pain. This can cause a pain problem for any of us.

A pain with a diagnosed cause, like a broken bone, could end up being a widespread pain coming from the central nervous system. This centralised pain can happen because having pain can aggravate our brain chemistry.

It is also possible for the pain to stay in one place but be *amplified* by the brain, which is another way to develop centralised pain.

Let's say in my town, five people broke their leg last month. Four of these people healed nicely and have no lasting pain. One of those five seemed fine too, their bone healed and their leg was fine to walk on, but they still felt some pain. It is likely for this person that their brain and nervous system have become a bit muddled and their pain now has a centralised origin.

Pain experts now think that a proportion of all chronic pain is centralised[1].

This all means that if your pain started:

- from an injury,
- from a surgery,
- with fatigue and aches,
- or a combination of these.

And if your pain has continued beyond three months, then current scientific evidence says you have probably developed centralised pain. It also says that if you have ongoing pain from a structural problem (like arthritis or an old injury), then *some* of your pain is also now a centralised type pain.

Fibromyalgia pain

To be clear, the pain in fibromyalgia is coming from a central sensitisation in the brain. This type of pain is called centralised pain, neurogenic pain, or just 'brain pain'.

In this book I will not be looking at trapped nerves or joint problems, I am going to concentrate on this neurogenic or 'brain pain' coming from the central nervous system because there are very few books that explain what we can do about it.

Centralised or 'brain pain' is the type of pain we will be exploring in this book.

I want to say something important before we explore further because, whatever you have been told, and whatever may have been implied about your condition, you are not responsible for creating it.

There is absolutely no blame or shame in having this condition.

There is plenty of knowledge about biological functions that can explain chronic pain and fibromyalgia but, surprisingly, is not readily available to patients.

There *are* routes out of fibromyalgia, and some that may require you to make lifestyle and diet changes. But at no point do any of these suggestions imply you have caused the illness. I want to give you all the information that I have found, to help you to get yourself out of a fibromyalgia or chronic pain state.

EXPLORING PAIN

1

THE CHEMICALS BETWEEN US

Before we explore *why* we might develop a chronic pain state like fibromyalgia, and how we can treat it, I'd like to talk to you about prescription pain killers.

The path that I recommend, in order to move away from the fibromyalgia state, discourages relying on pain killers. But I'd like you to understand why.

Current treatments for fibromyalgia

Continuing our tour of pain, we'll explore some simple chemistry, so that we can understand why certain medical drugs are prescribed for fibromyalgia.

There are many chemicals in the body that can be out of balance during fibromyalgia (things like *Substance P*, yes that is its name) but I am going to focus on 'glutamate'. Firstly, because it is the most abundant neurotransmitter in the brain, and secondly because glutamate is significant in *all* chronic pain patterns, and especially in fibromyalgia.

If you have ever been given pregabalin or gabapentin then you have experienced adjusting the levels of glutamate in your brain. Even if you haven't ever used these drugs it will help to know a little about what glutamate does.

Glutamate

The science part: Glutamate is a naturally occurring amino acid (part of a protein molecule) and it functions as a neurotransmitter in the brain and spinal cord. A neurotransmitter is a chemical that is used by the nerves to transmit information from one nerve cell to another nerve cell.

After glutamate is used to transmit signals across the nerve synapses (junctions) it is then changed into glutamine (another protein), before being recycled back into glutamate to be used again. Glutamate is a completely normal brain chemical and the brain needs it for many essential processes.

Need to know: Glutamate tends to *increase* neural signals in the brain and makes the brain cells fire more rapidly.

If you prefer to imagine your brain is like a car, then increasing glutamate is like putting your foot on the accelerator, adding more fuel to the engine and increasing the speed of the car. But if your car drives too fast you can get into problems. Things get overheated and the car's engine doesn't work so well. There is also a safe speed range that the brain should operate within, so too much glutamate is a problem. For example we know that:

- An increase in glutamate is regarded as a reason that pain feelings are amplified[1].
- Increased levels of glutamate are seen in the brains of people with fibromyalgia[2], and are associated with chronic pain.
- Abnormal levels of glutamate are also found in people with

most mental illnesses. This includes Bipolar Disorder, Obsessive Compulsive Disorder, and depression[3].

- Acute stress and inflammation can increase the glutamate levels in the brain and spinal cord[4].
- Glutamate levels in the body are often higher in people with cancer.

When abnormally high levels of glutamate are present, the brain starts to 'wind-up'. The brain gets faster and it can set off a cascade of signals that can become self-sustaining, like a feedback loop. This is like a car going so fast that it can't stop, and it runs through traffic lights and sets off all kinds of other warning systems.

Too much glutamate

We can prove the connection between glutamate and fibromyalgia because it's actually possible to *create* fibromyalgia! In animal studies, if glutamate was injected into the specific part of the brain that deals with how the body feels (the insular cortex), the injection exactly created fibromyalgia-like symptoms, including peripheral pain and increased sensitivity to touch and temperature[5].

Glutamate outside of the brain

The science part: the blood in the body and the blood in the brain do not mix directly. Substances moving from one side to the other have to pass a barrier called the blood-brain-barrier. It's a bit like immigration control at an airport, but for your brain.

Glutamate is also used as a signalling chemical outside of the brain for our body systems. We have receptors for glutamate in the cells of *all* of our major organ systems and also in our immune system cells, our skin, connective tissue, bones, and muscle cells. There is about 40 times as much glutamate in the blood circulating around our body as there is in the brain.

Need to know: In the body, glutamate is known as an *immuno-transmitter*, which means it's also a substance the body uses to move messages between the immune system and the nervous system[6].

I'm giving you a lot of information about glutamate because it is a really important body chemical in pain conditions, *and we have some control over it.*

- Glutamate takes a leading role in transmitting sensory information from the body to the brain. (We will see how this is important, later when we look at digestion).
- Glutamate in our blood can rise by 300% as a result of oxidative stress, which is a kind of stress on the body mainly caused by eating poor-quality food.[7]
- Glutamate is an irritant to brain cells and can actually kill individual cells if the levels are too high, creating inflammation in the brain (neuro-inflammation).

Drugs and glutamate

Many medications given for fibromyalgia and pain are drugs that block the receptor sites on nerve cells that glutamate would attach to in the brain and spinal cord (the central nervous system) which stops glutamate acting on those nerve cells. In our car analogy this would be like changing the fuel injection settings so that less fuel gets into the engine and it can't go so fast.

One of these types of drugs is the *NMDA* (N-methyl-D-aspartate) *receptor antagonists*. The drugs pregabalin (brand name; Lyrica), gabapentin, ketamine and tramadol belong to this category.

The idea is that by blocking the glutamate uptake in our brain and spinal cord cells, pain levels will decrease. In studies on rats and mice this is generally the case and so these drugs are prescribed for chronic widespread pain in humans.

[Interestingly, the vitamins magnesium and zinc also act as natural glutamate blockers.]

That's good news for rats... but what about for humans?

A rat might be relieved that his pain has gone, but he's not as complicated as a human being and he can't tell us if he feels completely ok on those drugs. The problem for humans is that glutamate helps our brains perform many different functions. For instance, glutamate also allows us to learn and create memories.

Drugs that interrupt glutamate in the brain might relieve some pain by blocking brain activity in these cells but in humans they also tend to have unpleasant side effects including nausea, anxiety, and hallucinations.

Glutamate-blocking drugs are also not especially effective at reducing the pain[8]. The Cochrane report found that only one in ten people given pregabalin (Lyrica) had good results, and found it was able to half their pain (that was the best result), while eight out of ten people suffered side effects while taking it[9]. Pregabalin (Lyrica) isn't even licensed for fibromyalgia in Europe or the UK as the results of the trials in Europe were so poor.

The biggest problem for patients, however, is that these drugs do nothing to resolve the original *cause* of the condition, which means they are expected to keep taking these drugs indefinitely.

Many people find they develop a tolerance to the drugs they are prescribed, so they have to keep increasing their dose, sometimes over several years. Eventually, they reach a threshold where they cannot safely take a higher dose.

So, glutamate plays an important role in our body's processing of pain signals. And taking drugs to reduce glutamate is one possibility in treating fibromyalgia, but what if we could find other ways to reduce it?

As we continue, I will show you some triggers that cause the body to increase glutamate. By understanding these triggers, and then doing something differently, we will be able to prevent these increases and start to take control of fibromyalgia.

I have deliberately avoided talking about opioid drugs so far. These are drugs such as oxycodone, fentanyl, buprenorphine, methadone, oxymorphone, hydrocodone, codeine, and morphine, and that's because these drugs can actually make pain worse.

I will explain why opioids are not helpful for chronic pain later on but our next step is to look at what stressful events can do to our bodies.

2

STRESSED OUT

Stress... and pain

People with fibromyalgia:

- show a higher stress response,
- have more internal sensitivity to sensations,
- and have a higher autonomic nervous system reactivity[1].

This means that they respond to stress more quickly and more easily.

What is stress?

At times in our lives we might be working hard or be 'run-down' and tired. We might find that our sleep is impacted and our digestion isn't so good. We are usually aware of this feeling and call it 'stress'.

If we have a fearful or painful experience, our autonomic nervous system will try and help, to prevent this happening again. To help us avoid experiencing similar situations in the future it often makes us more alert and vigilant. This hyperalertness can become an ongoing response to stress.

What does stress do to us?

Ongoing stress can make actual changes happen in our body's architecture. Physical changes that are possible from chronic or repeated stress:

- Our blood vessels may change their routes.
- Our lymphatic vessels can become dilated and change their flow rates.
- Nerves can grow, shrink or change routes.
- Parts of our brain can shrink and become smaller.
- Receptors on brain cells can change, altering brain chemistry[2].
- The immune system is not as effective during stress.
- The mucus in our gut reduces, and this leaves the gut vulnerable.

One study looked at children who had previously experienced a relocation when their family moved house, and found that they had more *gut permeability*. Gut permeability isn't a good thing, as it means some molecules that should remain in the gut can escape into the blood, and end up where they shouldn't be[3]. These children showed a higher chance of having allergies due to gut permeability, all caused by the stress of moving house.

We can demonstrate that stress affects our chemistry. One study in a London hospital did tests on people to see what happened to their blood chemistry after a stressful event. A 'stress test' was created by giving them an IQ test to do in 50 minutes (which should really take an hour), while playing different kinds of music in each ear (folk and rock music). The test candidates had reminders to hurry up and finish, and people kept coming in every fifteen minutes to check their blood pressure. Thirty minutes after finishing the stress test a particularly nasty inflammatory chemical, called TNF-alpha, showed an increase of over 100%, which is very significant, and a 54% increase in their level of IL-6,[4] (another inflammatory chemical).

These studies show us that stress increased participants' internal levels of inflammation.

Fortunately, most of the changes that happen due to stress are fully reversible when we relax and make changes to our lives!

Organisation between the body and brain

Your body wants to be looked after, that's the basics of it. It wants to be fed, watered, cleaned, rested, to feel safe, to be exercised and to relax.

It might be useful (and more fun) if we imagine that each of our bodies is an organisation. We operate as mobile businesses, and the primary focus of our businesses is harvesting (eating) and energy production (so we can find the next meal), along with some small-scale farming (of gut bacteria) in our large intestines.

You could imagine your cells as mini departments that produce energy. Cells hang out in groups where they make up the different body organs, beautifully specialised to perform a different task.

The lungs take oxygen from the air, and the kidneys are busy filtering blood. Our skin is the outer membrane around us that we can see, and inside us is the fascia; a set of thin stretchy bags around each of our organs, muscles, and body parts that keeps them separated.

All of these different organ systems need to know what everyone else is doing, just like different departments within an organisation, so really good internal communication systems are needed.

The nervous system acts as a communication system between the different organ departments and, to help you understand how it works, I'm going to give each part of the nervous system a job in our energy production company (body).

There is the brain and spinal cord (these two are called the *central nervous system*) who are the managing director (brain) and the board of directors (spinal cord).

Then there are three other groups of nerves in the body; the journalists, the movement people, and the autonomic lot who – as in many organisations – tend to get on with all of the less obvious but very important jobs and get ignored a bit.

The journalists (your sensory nerves) write reports to send to the brain, and they are interested in sensations. There are three different types of journalist. There are mechanical journalists who send reports about pressure, maybe like something touching your arm. Then there are chemical journalists who send reports to the brain about things that sting, like acids or salt in a skin wound. Finally, temperature journalists check on the internal weather and tell the brain if body parts are hot, cold, or nicely comfortable.

The movement people (the motor nerves) take signals from the brain and spinal cord to make the body move, which helps the body get to its' next meal.

And finally, there are a group of employees running an automated system that never stops (the autonomic nervous system). They run all the things that need to be kept going all of the time, like your heartbeat, your breathing, your digestion, or liver function etc.

There are other communication systems in the body too, like the endocrine system, which delivers mail in the body. The chemical employees have a series of glands that also help with communication, but they do it with hormone messages.

Office politics

Your brain has a penthouse office at the top of this organisation with a hard, bony covering to keep it safe, and it has been given the job of look-out. It's got the eyes and ears up there... but the brain's main job is to make sense of what the body it telling it. The brain receives a huge number of little messages from the body, and it turns each of these messages into either a 'thought' or a 'feeling'.

As a body owner, our usual tendency is to position 'me', my personality, as the director, in the brain, and the body just becomes an apparatus to move 'me' and my brain about.

Thinking this way causes no obvious problems, except that the body is not signed up to this version of events.

This is pretty much the same situation as in most actual human businesses!

Management think the company is theirs, but the employees know the company only exists because they make it happen.

Talent management

In real human organisations and companies, old fashioned managing directors might think that they are in charge of a group of people who are paid to run things for their (the director's) benefit. Even if the MD, board of directors, or shareholders would not openly admit to this ideology, many companies operate as if this is what they *do* believe.

Most employees, on the other hand, tend to feel that the organisation is made from their hard work and that it should support them in their employment, beyond just paying them. The organisation should, at the very least, provide a safe and secure working environment and preferably provide perks, benefits, and incentives.

Without these things, the employees are likely to complain continually or even go on strike.

In many human organisations *most* communication goes from the director down to the employees via management, with only minimal information going back up the other way. If you have ever worked at the bottom of an organisation, say as a receptionist or administrator, did the director ever *personally* ask you how your job was or if you had any ideas about how the whole organisation could be improved?

[If your company uses a Japanese management system then you may be able to answer 'yes' to this question, otherwise the majority of us have to answer 'no'.]

In the body, however, the director *does* have to listen. Those automatic nervous system employees have a hotline straight to the brain. They have an expansive communication system that takes masses of reports and feedback *up* to the brain. And the nerve they use to get it all up there is the vagus nerve, which is linked to all of our internal organs.

The vagus nerve is the largest nerve in the body after the spinal cord, and only 20% of the information it carries is instructions from the brain *down* to the internal organs, whereas 80% is information coming from those automatic nervous system employees and is going *up* to the brain.

As far as the body is concerned, the brain (including the mind and personality) exist to service and look after the body, not the other way round.

As we delve further into how the body gets out of balance, and how chronic pain states like fibromyalgia can develop, looking at the world from the position of the *body*, will help things start to make sense.

Special delivery

The reason for taking a tour of our nervous system was to get a grip on how the autonomic nervous system, running all our internal organs, communicates *directly* with the brain. Not all nerves have this special relationship.

The journalists we met, the sensory, mechanical, and temperature nerves, don't have this hotline to the brain. Instead they have to report to the spinal cord, and the spinal cord relays some of the messages to the brain. Some instructions for the body can also come directly from the spinal cord, rather than bother the brain with too many details.

The brain also doesn't get consulted about some emergency situations. If you put your hand on a hot stove your thermal journalists will report to the spinal cord and the spinal cord sends orders to the motor nerves to get your hand off the stove immediately. They don't bother to consult with the brain first, because by that time you'd have burned yourself.

State of me

One of our autonomic nerves is the vagus nerve, which is also described as a cranial nerve.

The cranial nerves go directly into the brain, they don't go via the spinal cord and they mainly act to control the face and skull areas. However, the route of the vagus nerve is rather different to the others.

The vagus nerve runs from the base of the skull, around our ears, then down the sides of our neck, and all the way down inside the body to reach almost all of our internal body organs.

The vagus nerve helps the body achieve '*homeostasis*' , which just means *internal balance*. By telling the brain, about how our internal organs are doing, other body systems can respond and adjust to each other.

If one day our intestines aren't feeling so comfortable, maybe because they didn't appreciate the kind of food we ate the day before, the intestines can send signals up to the brain via the vagus nerve. The brain receives and processes that information, so that the legs can be instructed to take the body away from the pizza parlour today and towards the salad bar instead.

So, the brain listens to the body and interprets the signals it receives. Then the brain sends out messages in order to regulate what is happening. This is normal and happens in everyone's body.

If one day I am late for a meeting and I see my friend walking a distance ahead of me, my brain and my autonomic nervous system can co-ordinate my body's response to increase my breathing and heart rate, so that I am ready to run and catch them up. The brain and body are designed to listen to each other and to co-ordinate themselves so that everything happens seamlessly.

Using our vagus nerve as a tool

So, the vagus nerve is an information highway, which is all very interesting, but the reason I'm telling you about it is because we can use this information *practically* in the treatment of chronic pain. You see, we are able hijack this clever system; we can get the vagus nerve to send signals that *we choose* to our brain!

It's like being able to get into the email account from the automatic nervous system employees and send extra emails from their account up to the brain.

If we actively do things with our body like a slow breathing exercise, for instance, we can fool the brain and nervous system. Breathing deep slow breaths is normally a signal that the body is relaxed, so – if we breathe like this – our automatic nervous system employees use the vagus nerve and dutifully transmit an '*everything down here is relaxed*' message up to the brain.

We tend to think that the brain is always in charge, but actually the brain responds to what the body feels, much more than we are aware of. This is how our digestion affects our mood, and how physical damage can create depression. In fact, all of our emotions are actually based on how our body *feels* and the messages it sends to our brain.

Putting on a face

One well-known way you can fool your brain is to hold a pencil sideways in your mouth. When you hold the pencil between your teeth like this it creates a kind of a smile, by stretching the mouth. Even this fake smile has been shown to have an effect on our mood. The brain believes we are happier as we are apparently smiling, and it aligns itself with this idea. Our brain chemistry changes because of the body movement (the fake smile in this instance).

Botox is used by some people to paralyze their frown muscles between the eyes, and this paralysis can actually help those people to feel more relaxed. When the face seems calm, the brain assumes that we are calm in our environment and therefore we must be ok. I should say, though, that we can get this effect naturally just by reminding ourselves to relax our face and smile more often!

It should also be noted that Botox users who totally disable the muscles around their mouth or eyes may be inadvertently telling their brains that they *cannot* smile fully anymore, therefore giving their brains a rather less optimistic impression of the world!

Charles Darwin was the first to realise that we all use the same facial expressions all over the world. He travelled all over the globe to check that this was true and he realised that we respond to our environment instinctively, without thinking. Poker players especially know it can be hard to stop ourselves revealing our feelings this way. The brain sometimes only gets told what we felt *after* we have physically responded, although this is so fast that we don't notice the order in which it happens.

Give it a try: smile and relax your forehead and brow muscles. Even if you don't *feel* especially happy it will still help your body chemistry.

Stress and the vagus nerve

Stress effects

Our autonomic nervous system is divided into two main parts. Let's say that the autonomic nervous system has two teams of employees, called the sympathetic team and parasympathetic team, and these teams of nerves respond automatically to our environment for us, without our awareness.

The parasympathetic team is the 'zen' team; they help our body to relax and feel calm. (The vagus nerve is on this team).

The sympathetic team gets us motivated, hyped-up, alert, angry, twitchy or ready to run away.

> I remember which-is-which by thinking of a parachute, which is a safe, going-down kind of a thing, and that we might feel 'sympathetic' or sorry for ourselves if we are angry and stressed out.

These two ANS teams can produce a wide range of responses to our environment. They take us from feeling calm and safe, all the way over to feeling extremely threatened and fearful. I imagine they operate by having a tug of war, so one team can pull the system one way, and then the other team pulls it the other way.

These teams should happily push and pull us back and forth from being stressed or needing to move fast (if something happens that we need to respond to, like being late and being in a rush to get to work) to then relaxing us again when the stress is over (we can sit quietly again).

If our body is always on alert, then the sympathetic nervous team is always pulling and our calming parasympathetic team (along with the vagus nerve) gets deactivated and doesn't pull.

If we are on edge or hyperalert like this for too long, the elevated level of alertness can start to negatively affect how our vagus nerve is actually functioning. A properly functioning vagus nerve (that allows us to feel calm) is said to have 'vagal tone' – in the same way we might say someone who is fit and active is 'toned'.

If the sympathetic team are always winning and pulling the system towards alertness, then our parasympathetic (zen) team doesn't do very much. If the vagus nerve was a person then it would be getting unfit and flabby.

If an 'alert' state continues then the 'tone' of the vagus nerve gets reduced.

If we remain stressed for *really* prolonged periods then the whole system can simply get stuck in one place, and it usually gets stuck in an alert, ready to run, kind of state.

Stress can be difficult to measure because it affects lots of body processes. However, because the vagus nerve carries information about stressful events in the body (like that pizza), we can use it to measure our response to stress. (Eating badly is also a kind of stress for the body, just like rushing about all the time.)

What's significant about low vagal tone?

Unfortunately, low vagal tone is not a healthy thing for humans to live with. We know that "*decreased vagal function is associated with an increased risk for morbidity and mortality*"[5]. Low vagal tone is also associated with a slowing of our prefrontal brain activity and with immune dysfunction.

Can we measure our vagal tone?

Yes. Rather than measure the functioning of a nerve, which is difficult to get at while you are using it, it is easier to measure one thing that the vagal nerve regulates.

One result of having *low* vagal tone, when the vagus nerve is not functioning well, is low 'heart rate variability' (HRV). This is because the brain and heart are connected by the vagus nerve.

We can use HRV as a measure of vagal tone, and this is a really easy thing for us to measure. If you have a smartphone you can buy an app that can measure it from your finger, using the phone's camera.

What is heart rate variability (HRV)?

Our heartbeats are not all completely equal. Our heart rate will naturally speed up a little, and then slow down a little, in response to how much the body needs it to, even while we just sit still. We tend to think that our heartbeats should be regular, but in fact this slight variation is regarded as a signal of good health[6].

Basically, more variability is a good thing, because it shows our system is flexible.

Heart rate variability (HRV) gives an indication of our body's ability to self-stabilize in response to stress.

If the body doesn't respond adaptively to stressful events, then the heartbeats stay in a more regular pattern. This is a heart with low variability.

In tests, people with low HRV are much more likely to show increased startle response to a loud noise[7], which means they are more easily shocked and scared.

Low HRV (low vagal tone) is associated with several more serious things that we would all like to avoid, like:

- A reduced resilience to stress
- Depression
- Anxiety
- Cardiovascular disease
- Higher blood glucose levels
- Immune dysfunction
- Inflammation

Low vagal tone is also associated with poor self-regulation, less behavioural flexibility, and anxiety disorders.

So, we can use our heartbeats to see how the vagus nerve is doing. HRV allows us to measure *how* stressed the body is feeling:

Good vagal tone (that allows calm feelings) = Good HRV (ability to deal with stress)

Low vagal tone (poorly functioning vagus nerve) = _Low_ HRV (poor response to stress)

HRV and fibromyalgia

Low heart rate variability is very common in people with fibromyalgia[8]. In fact, people with fibromyalgia are *so likely* to have a low HRV that HRV has been proposed as a 'bio-marker' for fibromyalgia. A bio-marker is a clinical sign that could be used as a diagnostic criteria for the condition[9].

Your HRV should be within a certain range for your age and gender[10]. You can download fitness apps that can measure your HRV on a smartphone so you can see your score and track improvements in your HRV over time.

Are there other connections between the vagus nerve, fibromyalgia, and pain?

Yes, lots. The vagus nerve controls the mechanisms by which serotonin is released from the small intestine[11]. Serotonin is a very important brain chemical that allows us to feel happy. Serotonin also helps the body to know when we are feeling full after eating and it aids gut movement. Alterations in serotonin levels can cause disruption in the wake-sleep cycle, cause depression and anxiety, and increase our pain sensitivity.

The vagus nerve also has the ability to inhibit thalmic 'pain' pathways at the spinal cord[12]. These are generally regarded as the main pathways that indicate warnings of damage to the central nervous system.

The vagus nerve helps our digestion to work properly. When we are relaxed, the vagus nerve increases our digestive enzymes to break down our food. It lowers our blood pressure and it helps to regulate the immune system.

Good vagal tone is associated with us having more efficient blood glucose regulation, which helps to lower the risk of diabetes, stroke and cardiovascular disease.

Vagal nerve stimulation has been shown to protect the gut from the effects of stress in animals. This means that the vagus nerve may be able to protect us from the effects of stress, and improving the function of the vagus nerve may be able to reverse the negative effects that stress has on our digestion[13].

Need to know - vagus nerve facts

- The vagus nerve is part of our parasympathetic nervous system (the calming part).
- The vagus nerve takes information from the body *up* to the brain.
- We can hijack these signals to send our own messages to the brain, for instance by using body movements.
- We can use the vagus nerve to measure our ability to manage stress (via HRV).
- The vagus nerve needs to work well for good health.
- The vagus nerve is very much connected with our digestion.
- The vagus nerve can get 'unfit' and lack tone, which means its isn't working as well to calm us down.

The vagus nerve is *so* interesting that a group of scientists started running electrical currents up it to the brain to see what happened next!

Vagal nerve stimulation

The scientists who invented a vagal nerve stimulator were actually trying to work out how a chemical, that they had injected into the brain of a rat, had lowered inflammation levels in the body of that rat. The chemical they had used couldn't get out of the brain, so the signal to turn off inflammation in the body was not chemical. This was not supposed to happen. They took out of the rat all of the obvious things that could have transmitted the signal with no success… until they took out the rat's vagus nerve, and then that effect didn't happen.

This proved that it was the vagus nerve that was telling the body to turn down the inflammation. The vagus nerve can't move chemicals, so the scientists started experimenting with ways they could somehow stimulate the vagus nerve to reduce inflammation, and one method that worked was with electricity.

They developed a medical device called a Vagal Nerve Stimulator (VNS), which is a small device that can be implanted inside someone's neck to electrically stimulate the vagus nerve, and it is now licensed to treat rheumatoid arthritis, MS and epilepsy[14].

What this research proves to us with fibromyalgia is that the vagus nerve has extraordinary control over inflammation in the body. If the vagus nerve is surgically removed it leads to increased inflammation in the body.

Bioelectric medicine

Electrical stimulators for the vagus nerve are now also used on the outside of the skin and have been shown to reduce glutamate levels[15]. This indicates that increasing vagal tone can reduce glutamate levels and reduce inflammation.

Other cranial nerves are also being targeted, with new electrical devices that fit under the tongue to create 'neuro-modulation', which means making the brain re-route its signals and create new paths. This can help with the after effects of stroke or brain damage, where part of the brain has died and new brain connections are needed.

However, giving our nerves electric shocks isn't entirely comfortable, plus some of the devices need to be used for hours, creating skin discomfort and irritation.

Research for fibromyalgia

Bioelectric devices don't treat fibromyalgia but I am telling you about this new bioelectric medicine because it has produced lots of new research about the vagus nerve and other cranial nerves, which demonstrates that these nerves have a huge effect on the brain's control over the body.

Fortunately, there are much safer and less expensive options that we can use at home to tone our vagus nerve.

Information we can use

The acupressure points that I found to help with fibromyalgia symptoms are all around the neck. Many of them are directly over the vagus nerve and other cranial nerves in the neck area. This is where ancient acupuncture theories connect with western medical science to create a natural pain treatment system. And it is what I'm most excited about in regards to finding effective treatments for fibromyalgia and chronic pain.

It is the vagus nerve's job to respond to the levels of inflammatory chemicals in our blood and turn off their production. The fibres of the vagus nerve can sense *cytokines*, which are an important inflammation chemical.

Inflammation is a critical problem in fibromyalgia and we can use this information about the vagus nerve to help us.

As we continue, we will be looking at how to keep our vagus nerve in good working order. We'll see how the vagus nerve is an important tool for unravelling the fibromyalgia condition because of its key role in communicating between the body and the brain.

The next chapter unravels how traumatic events can influence the development of fibromyalgia, and how the vagus nerve is involved here too.

FIBROMYALGIA AND THE AUTONOMIC NERVOUS SYSTEM (ANS)

3

TRAUMA AND FIBROMYALGIA

In this chapter, we'll find out how past experiences of fear and trauma may have affected your autonomic nervous functions, and how these experiences could be continuing to impact your physical health. Even if you have not experienced events like this it is worth knowing that long-term stress or hard work can push the body into physical states using the processes explained in this chapter.

Early life adversity is strongly associated with fibromyalgia, as well as with many other illnesses later in life but, interestingly, early life adversity is experienced by many more people with *physical* illnesses than with mental illnesses[1]. This is due to the way that our autonomic nervous system alters the way our body works.

The Polyvagal theory

The Polyvagal theory, published by Dr. Porges in 1995, describes the way the autonomic nervous system moves our body through different responses, without us being conscious of it doing so.

We feel the physical changes in our body. For instance, if we are nervous we might feel our palms are clammy or notice an increase in our heart rate.

Our tug-of-war teams, the parasympathetic and sympathetic (our autonomic nervous system), are designed to move us smoothly through a normal range of body states in response to our environment. They will automatically return us to a calm state, which is the only place our digestion works really well, when we are safe.

The modern model of our autonomic nervous system[2] describes a wide range of possible states; from feeling safe to being terrified[3].

The table below demonstrates these states.

Faint	***Shut-down (surrender)***	***Fright - Fight***	***Flight or Play***	***Alert!*** **(Observe and check)**	***Rest & Digest***
Abnormal/Emergency responses		Emergency response	Normal range of Autonomic Nervous System responses		
Loss of consciousness	Frozen with fear	Ready for action but also fearful	Body gets ready for action	Attentive, watchful	Calm, feeling safe
Faint: extreme fear with flaccid immobility. Low blood pressure and heart rate slowing causing loss of consciousness (vasovagal syncope)	Heart rate slows Blood pressure lowers Blood vessels to the skin dilate Pain numbed Cognitive failure and emotional numbing Withdrawl of pro-social behaviours,. Might show a blank expression, mono-tone voice and avoid eye contact	Similar to *Flight or Play* but with more emotional arousal or more fear.	Adrenaline secreated Heart rate increases Sweating increases Vagal tone reduced Digestion is inhibited Bronchiooles of the lung dilate allowing easier oxygen uptake Pupils dilate allowing more light to enter the eye for distance vision.	Lowered heart rate, followed by cardiac acceleration (faster heart rate) If there is a threat the body continues to prepare for *Flight-Play.* If there is no threat the body returns to *Rest & Digest*	Blood vessels leading to the gut dilate, allowing more blood flow. Salivary gland secretion is stimulated Peristalsis is accelerated (gut movement) Constriction of the pupil allows for closer vision

In the alert and mobilised states, where we can run away, (*Fright, Fight* and *Flight or Play*), the body is told by the sympathetic team to send extra blood to our muscles and to activate sweating, so that we can cool down if we are about to run and move.

You may be wondering why '*Play*' is on the list. *Play & Sports* can be a mobilised, high-alert state but it is usually without fear.

The final options of *Shut-Down* or *Faint* (pass out from fear) are not in our normal range of responses. These are emergency defence options to help us to survive a life-threatening situation.

In the temporary *Shut-Down* (surrender) state, the sympathetic team is afraid for our life and does not believe that running away is possible or safe. Rather than risk dying by fighting with a stronger predator, instead we surrender and play dead, so we can recover and get away when the danger has passed.

Any event in which we are scared, and cannot move ourselves out of the danger, can trigger a defensive *Shut-Down* from the sympathetic team. The *Shut-Down* state can be triggered by violent events, abuse, emotional trauma, accidents, phobias, or surgery (even when we are under anaesthetic). One of the things that also happens in the *Shut-Down* state is that both our heart and our brain slow down, and we dissociate from our feelings, making us feel numb emotionally.

If we experience life threatening situations regularly, the sympathetic team and the body may learn to go into this state more often (maybe triggering a *Shut-Down* state even in less threatening events) because the dissociation effect in the brain can help us cope with intense fear and distress.

During long periods of stress, the body can reach a point where it feels it cannot deal with the environment it has to live in and begins to give up. We might also call this state 'burn-out', adrenal fatigue, nervous exhaustion, or a nervous breakdown.

It is also possible for the nervous system to get habituated in one mode of operating. The nervous system gets stuck in some of these states and does not return fully to the safe *Rest and Digest* state. This helps us to understand why trauma or stress can have such long lasting effects on our bodies.

This is how sustained stress and fear can become a *physical* problem.

Trauma does not need to necessarily include pain or physical harm. Studies show that just watching painful facial expressions can result in an increased pain sensitivity[4], which could affect children and adults who are exposed to violent environments.

After witnessing terrible events, some people who had been in a fearful situation or felt traumatised reported feeling cut off from their emotions or being unable to feel joy or love, indicating that their autonomic nervous system had not returned to *Rest and Digest*.

The changes that happen to the nervous system are on a cellular level and have been proven scientifically; these are not just woolly estimations. This is important information to correct the attitude of some medics about 'personality' being the root of fibromyalgia.

We can find a link between some of the known causes of fibromyalgia; like childhood trauma, acute stress or surgery, and the types of event that may cause a *Shut-Down* response from the autonomic nervous system. We can see from the table of bodily changes that the *Shut-Down* state has a slowed down metabolism and dampened emotions, and that it is a generally depressed state of being. This can be an effect of low vagal tone.

When our nervous system stays partially in *Shut-Down,* we cannot easily feel happiness or love, and this state is called 'dissociation'. We will return to the specific effects of dissociation later in the book.

Childhood events

Changes to the nervous system can happen to children whose brain and nervous system is still developing. Experiencing neglect, or living with someone with a mental illness or alcohol problem, are common causes of sustained fear and anxiety for children.

Early life adversity is also referred to as adverse childhood events (ACE).

The number of ACEs someone has experienced statistically correlates to their health later in life; the more ACEs the person has experienced the higher their chances are of developing an illness later in life.

Adverse childhood events (ACEs) include experiences like:

Infection, serious illness, stress, bullying, domestic violence, parental abandonment through separation or divorce, having a parent with a mental health condition, being the victim of abuse (physical, sexual or emotional), being neglected (physically or emotionally), having a member of the household being in prison, and growing up in a household where there are people with alcohol and drug problems.

Remembered stress - the science

It might seem obvious that the effects of stress or fear could impact us psychologically. We might expect that our thinking could be changed by difficult experiences when we are growing up, but we are now able to prove that ACEs can have physical effects on our brain and nervous system. (See the **Your Brain's Surveillance System** at the end of this chapter).

When the growing brain learns to be be prepared for fear and stress, it is learning to respond more quickly to those triggers. As an adult it takes less stress or fear to trigger the brain into a stressed or *Alert!* state.

These changes can also create depression, overturning the idea that all depression is caused by our thinking. Accidents, illnesses or just unreliable parenting can all have similar effects on the nervous system.

Fortunately our brains have the ability to heal and change, even as an adult, or after many years of difficulty. Understanding these processes can help to demystify the negative effects of ACEs and offer us ways to help each other.

Single stressful events

Even without any experience of childhood or adult trauma, we can prove that acutely stressful events can directly cause an increase of glutamate.

Rats that were restrained (to create acute stress) showed a release of glutamate[5]. Even more interestingly, after the rats had experienced this event their brains were altered. When these rats experienced another new stress event, they had a different response, and they responded to the second event with more anxiety-like and depressive behaviours. These new behaviours correlated with hyperactivity in the hippocampus area caused by the glutamate, and a reduction (down-regulation) in the receptors that normally control the release of glutamate (called the mGlu2 receptors).

So, by experiencing only one stressful event the rats' brains were less able to regulate glutamate during the second event.

For people, a single stressful event could be things like a serious illness, the loss of a loved one, a road-traffic accident, giving birth, having surgery, or any situation that was a shock to us.

Surrender or negotiate

According to the Poly Vagal theory, although the vagus nerve is part of the parasympathetic team (the calming team) it is also responsible for the *Faint* and *Shut-down* states. How?

This is something about the vagus nerve that was not often made clear but Dr. Porges usefully clarified this for us.

The vagus nerve has two strands. To stick with our idea of employees, there is one part of the vagus nerve that is really old (and uses some very out of date communication techniques) and another part that is much younger and up to date. These two employees both work in the parasympathetic (calming) tug of war team.

1)The old strand of the vagus (the dorsal vagus) controls the emergency *Shut-Down* and *Faint* (pass out) options.

This old (dorsal) strand of the vagus nerve was developed much earlier in our evolution when we were reptiles. Reptiles can stop breathing for long periods of time to avoid detection, so it was a very useful skill to stop breathing and play dead, but humans have evolved to be more complex than reptiles and if we stop breathing, and our heart rate slows too much, we simply pass out!

The dorsal vagus hasn't updated itself very much and still thinks the *Shut-Down* state is a good plan if things get too scary. This part of the vagus is like an employee that doesn't do discussion; if there is a problem, they just shut everything down and wait for something to change.

2) The younger strand (ventral) vagus controls what we would think of as normal, healthy relaxation and it allows us to be in *Rest and Digest.*

This relaxing (ventral) vagus calms our heart rate and it sends blood to the digestive system, so that we can get on with digesting our food. This part of the vagus nerve governs our voice, facial muscles, our heart, and our ears.

As a body employee, the ventral vagus would be in charge of social media. It helps us get on with other humans, assisting with communication and listening.

One notable function of this younger ventral vagus is that it can alter the way our ears work.

Hearing ourselves

In a relaxed state, we can most easily hear the middle spectrum of sounds, where human voices are pitched. When we move out of *Rest and Digest* into the mobilised *Alert!* States, the ear muscles are tightened so that we hear very high pitch sounds, like birds giving warning calls, and also very low vibrations.

The ventral vagus controls the tightening of the muscles around our ears.

This makes sense if we imagine our ancestors keeping a look out for tigers or other predators. When we were sitting about with other humans we listened to their voices, but when we got frightened we listened for birds calling out and maybe the sounds of animals running, making low vibrations in the ground.

It is very common to see ear problems in people with fibromyalgia, and it is often a vagus nerve symptom. Ear problems are something we regard as an early warning sign for fibromyalgia. In fact, when I see ear problems like muffled hearing, popping, clicking, or temporo-mandibular pain (TMJ) pain around the jaw, I always ask about stress and trauma in the person's history.

Listen to your heart

It is common to experience unpleasant chest symptoms with fibromyalgia. Some people experience chest pain, tightening of chest muscles, palpitations, racing heart, shaking inside, or dizziness. Our vagus nerve is in control of the heart, and specifically it controls the heart rate by a mechanism called the *vagal brake.*

The heart is actually set to run very fast but is kept to a slower speed by the vagus nerve; if we need the heart to start beating faster it is quicker to increase the heart rate by just removing the vagal brake. If we relied on the other mechanisms, we would have to wait for adrenaline to be secreted, travel in the blood to the heart, and then for the adrenaline to speed up our heart rate. This would be pretty quick, but not as quick as just removing the vagal brake.

When the ventral (young) vagus isn't working well, or we experience stress, the sympathetic team will pull the system over into activation and *Alert!*, and the vagal brake will be released. As the vagal brake is released, the heart is allowed to beat faster. If we need to run away from a tiger this might be useful, but if our stress is emotional we might experience uncomfortable physical sensations of fear and anxiety.

If the whole body is ready to run away and we are not running, the body can create an internal panic situation where we are breathing fast, our heartbeat is increased, and we are sweating (all sympathetic responses). The vagus nerve will have told the brain 'things are bad down here', so now the brain is getting fearful too. This is what we call a panic attack.

Vagal toning can teach our body to calm down again and to respond to stress differently. The body relearns the difference between wanting to run away and social anxiety.

And if our body responds to stress differently, we can notice a powerful effect on our pain levels.

Hard-wired social skills

Humans have developed skills to get along with each other. We can recognise facial expressions and voice tones to communicate our feelings with each other. Working together, in teams and tribes, has kept us safe and our nervous system has evolved to support this way of living.

The ventral (younger) vagus creates a strong connection between our sympathetic nervous system and our face muscles[6]. This allows us to look at another person and decide if they are in a calm state – are we safe to approach them? It also gives us the ability to indicate our state to other people too. Using our facial muscles in relation to other (safe to be with) humans uses this younger strand of the vagus nerve, and signals to our brain that we are in *Rest and Digest* rather than in *Alert!* (watching for tigers) mode.

When we feel good and are with people we like, we smile and our faces are relaxed. Our nervous system understands this and so it will relax our body into *Rest and Digest* mode.

Getting it all to work for us

The older *Shut-Down* mechanism is still within us, but should only be triggered as a last resort, as an emergency survival tool. The other sympathetic states, like *Fright or Fight* or *Alert,* are supposed to be temporary; we are not supposed to live permanently in these mobilised states. These states become 'stress' when we stay in them too long.

By using the vagus nerve as a messenger we can give our brain signals of calm and safety, which can encourage our body to spend more time in the relaxed *Rest and Digest* mode.

We've seen that the vagus nerve even has the power to reduce the kind of inflammation caused by rheumatoid arthritis, which is an auto-immune problem in the joints.

So, we want to calm our brain chemistry to reverse fibromyalgia, because calming the brain can reduce pain and clear the mind.

But how can we send calming messages to our brain?

- Actions that tell the brain that we are safe and happy, like relaxing our face and smiling.
- Activities that create cues of safety, like breathing deeply.
- Getting our gut and digestion to send messages to the brain that say 'everything is ok inside' with our diet.

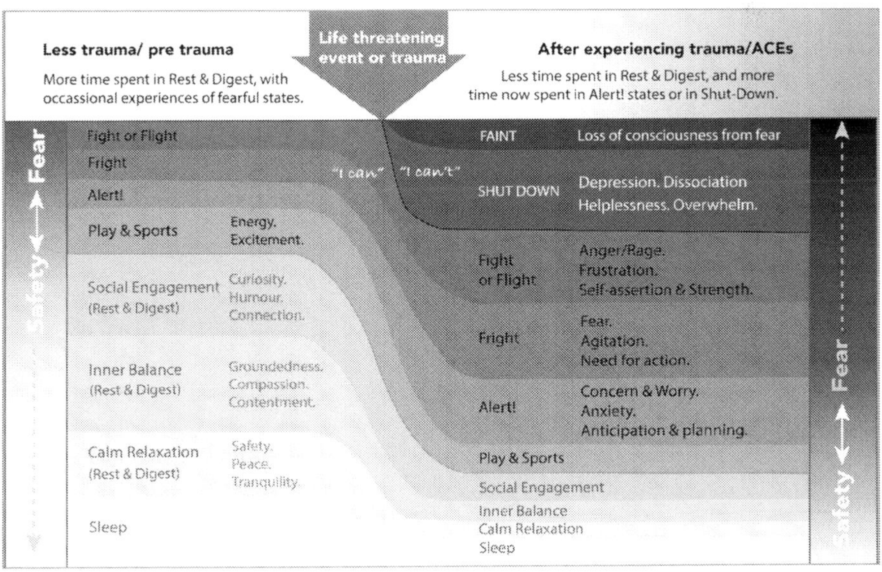

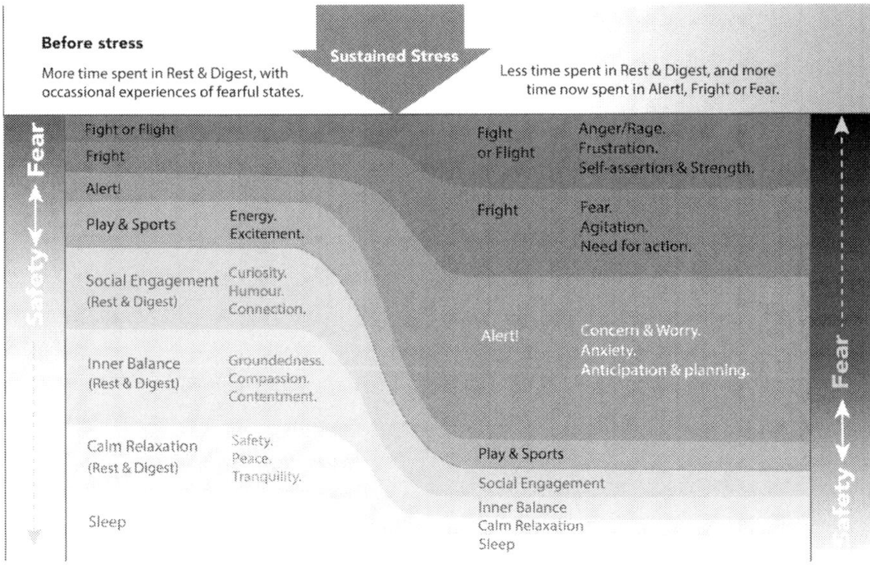

Moving on, with an understanding of your nervous system, we can now take a look at other triggers for fibromyalgia pain.

Your brain's surveillance system

For those of you who are interested I wanted to give you a bit more detail about how stress and trauma can affect the brain.

Our brains have a set of cells that act as a surveillance system, keeping watch over the whole brain. One of these types of cells are the *microglia* which are the immune cells in the brain. If the microglia cells detect inflammation, infection, or damage in the brain, they can change shape, and literally move themselves to that area of the brain and get busy clearing away the debris.

I like to think of the microglia as the undercover superheroes of our brain. When they are not active and rushing to an emergency, they act like gardeners in the brain. Microglia can stimulate new growth, helping with neuroplasticity, and they can also prune away cells that are damaged or old, which are then digested by the microglia. Microglia are either doing their day job as gardeners, or, if necessary they become activated and go to help with an emergency.

Another group of cells that work alongside the microglia cells are the *astrocytes*. Astrocytes aren't immune cells but they are involved with similar work to the microglia. Astrocytes also have two identities, and their normal 'day job' is to look after the chemistry between nerve endings.

At the end of every nerve there is a gap. Nerve are actually thin cells, like pieces of string, but instead of tying knots to join them all up, there is a gap at the ends called a synaptic gap. Nerves have to use a neurotransmitter, like glutamate, to transmit a signal across these gaps.

In your brain, each astrocyte is responsible for over 100,000 of these junctions and they monitor and adjust the chemistry in the synaptic gaps. Astrocytes are the caretakers for glutamate, they collect the glutamate and recycle it, so it can be used over and over again across the synaptic gaps. Re-uptake and recycling of glutamate by astrocytes is critical for preventing an excess of glutamate building up in the brain[7].

When there is an emergency in the brain these two cells work together. The microglia are the first to detect a problem and they become activated. They change their shape, and then move around the brain to get to the problem area. If necessary, the microglia can also send signals to tell the astrocytes to help them with the clean up.

Astrocytes can't move themselves but they are able to get extra help to come up to the brain from the body. Astrocytes look after and maintain the blood brain barrier (BBB), which is the sheet of cells keeping the brain safe from pathogens or infections, and keeping the brain separated from the body. When astrocytes are activated by signals from the microglia, the astrocytes can alter the BBB so it becomes more permeable, which allows extra immune cells to enter the brain from the body side.

Microglia tend to be early responders (within minutes) and then return promptly to their surveillance roles, whereas astrocytes are slower to activate but they are also slower to return to their protective state. Although repairing damage and inflammation are normal activities for both these cells, activated astrocytes and microglia have some unwanted effects, as they can also contribute to the development and persistence of chronic pain.

Activated astrocytes and microglia produce chemicals to reduce inflammation, but they are both also able to produce cytokines that *increase* inflammation, to signal to other cells that more help is needed on site. This means they might be signalling pro-inflammatory chemicals to get cells removed, and also signalling anti-inflammatory signals to keep this in check. The problem is that when there are many problems to deal with in the brain their sensitive chemical messaging can become chaotic and excessive.

Activated microglia produce the cytokine TNF-a which plays an important role in both starting and maintaining persistent pain and central sensitisation, and activated astrocytes release their glutamate, increasing the glutamate levels and increasing the sensations of pain[8].

Like most things in the body, small amounts of damage are easily repaired. However ongoing inflammation can cause problems for our repair cells, like the microglia and astrocytes who can end up always being in emergency clean-up mode, rather than repairing cells and creating regrowth.

The responsive brain

Our brain cells are not just automatic workers that we can forget about, they are sensitive to what we are doing in our lives.

Microglia are most active when we are sleeping. They are less active when we are awake. Microglia become less active when levels of noradrenaline (norepinephrine) in our body rise, and when noradrenaline levels are really high the microglia are actually unable to act and cannot repair damage at all[9].

This is how stress actually changes our brain chemistry. Noradrenaline (called norepinephrine in the USA) is a natural chemical that keeps us awake, but it is released in greater amounts when we are stressed or fearful. Noradrenaline moves our body from a *Rest & Digest* state, into the *Alert!* states and when our noradrenaline levels are high our microglia are disabled. Without our microglia functioning well to keep our brain healthy, we run the risk of increasing brain inflammation.

Stress hormones also reduce the number of astrocytes in the brain, and they reduce many of the astrocyte's critical functions that are needed for normal brain activity. When 'brain-fog' and poor concentration are such common symptoms in fibromyalgia we can see why finding ways to reduce our stress levels are so important, to keep our brains healthy.

Both acute episodes of stress, and chronic stress in adulthood, impair the recycling of glutamate by our astrocytes, which can lead to an increase in glutamate in the brain, and increase our pain sensitivity.

Astrocytes, like microglia, are also sensitive to an increase in other stress hormones (like our own natural corticosteriods) and these chemicals too can inhibit their function and impair synaptic transmission between brain cells.

In studies with young rats, daily separation from the mother (for three to four hours a day for two weeks) is enough to cause lasting reduction to astrocyte glutamate transporter function. Likewise, using noise as a stress has similar lasting effects, specifically reducing the glutamate recycling activities of astrocytes. These are not extreme forms of stress and yet they still show marked changes to the brain. Separated young rats are alone (although they can still see their parent) and potentially they experience being more vigilant, looking out for their own safety, and being attentive to potential threats. Remaining vigilant or fearful, and staying in *Alert!* states is not healthy for humans either because of these mechanisms in the brain.

In humans some of these types of research are too invasive (requiring multiple brain scans and brain biopsies), but newer, less invasive methods are becoming available to study the living brain. We are beginning to be able to prove how our human brains can be concretely affected by life events[10]. Recent studies indicate that early life adversity may 'prime' the responses of the astrocytes, so that people who have experienced early life adversity have a greater susceptibility to stress and disease states after a second stressful event later in life[11], just like rats.

Specifically, we also know that astrocytes and microglia play a key role in the creation and maintenance of chronic pain[12], which shows us how ACEs and chronic pain are linked in our brain.

All of this means that if you have experienced ACEs, or stress as an adult, your body may need a bit more help from you, in order to keep your stress levels low and stay healthy. Your system may not deal with stress as well as someone who had a safe and loving childhood, or someone who has not previously experienced a trauma. Fortunately our brains are very adaptable throughout our lives, and they can change and heal.

4

STRUCTURAL CAUSES

Sometimes fibromyalgia and chronic pain are not related to childhood trauma or high emotions. Physical or emotional trauma can force the body into a distressed state from fear, but it is also possible to push the body into a distressed state gradually over a period of time from several other causes.

Very frequently, people with fibromyalgia have worked hard or have pushed themselves to achieve a lot. They may have taken on too much or been under pressure. If they experienced difficulties or injury, they may have continued to work beyond what their bodies could manage.

Working hard for long periods, maybe skipping meals or managing on minimal sleep and resting, forces the body to remain in *Alert!* states. For these people, the sympathetic team in the autonomic nervous system is always pulling the body functions in the *Alert!* directions, which prevents repairs being made.

Body repairs can only be done in the relaxed states of *Rest and Digest* and *Sleep* and so small areas of damage can accumulate over time, giving multiple warning signals to the brain.

Stress becomes a long-term illness for the body. Repairs are not made, and a stress chemical called cortisol remains elevated, and inflammation levels rise. The body can maintain this state for short periods as a survival mechanism but if we live like this for long periods, we risk the body processes going wrong.

Fibromyalgia has a gradual onset. It does not appear overnight but can develop as the body becomes unbalanced. It is quite possible to have mild symptoms of fibromyalgia, or only have the pains in certain areas of the body, for many years.

Fatigue can be seen as a signal from the body that it needs to slow down and repair itself. The kind of resting where we are immobile on the sofa or bed is one way to rest but in clinic we find that stationary forms of resting need to be used along with gentle movement, mind-calming, and improvements to diet to reverse a fibromyalgia state.

Chronic pain can also occur after physical injuries, accidents, and surgery. In this section we will explore some common structural aspects that can affect fibromyalgia.

Surgery and fibromyalgia

It is well known that surgery is a common 'trigger' for fibromyalgia. It is very likely that people who develop fibromyalgia after surgery are already slightly out of balance from stress, or other factors like diet or lack of movement. The stressed body experiences the surgery as physical damage and yet more evidence that the environment is dangerous.

Professor Wolfe, a fibromyalgia specialist in the USA, proposes that every surgery patient should be assessed for FM-ness, to see how many fibromyalgia symptoms they might have, because it has been found that having even mild fibromyalgia-type symptoms decreases the effectiveness of surgery to relieve pain.

Even though, personally, we may want the surgery, and it might even be lifesaving, our autonomic nervous system knows nothing about it until we are immobilised and the surgeon cuts us. Our body experiences the surgery while our conscious personality is comfortably anaesthetised.

We rarely consider it, but our autonomic nervous system is still active in surgery. The job of the anaesthetist is to balance us carefully so that our conscious mind is not aware. At the same time, the anaesthetist must make sure that the autonomic nervous system is active, keeping our heart beating, our blood pressure stable, and our breathing regular. If there was too much anaesthetic in our system, the autonomic nervous system would also shut down and we would die. This delicate balance allows us to have surgery and remain safe, but we should remember that our body experiences the surgery.

Injuries from accidents or surgery often cause nerve damage, which heals quite quickly. However, sometimes an injury leaves scarring that creates tiny warning signals to be sent to the brain, even after the area is completely healed. These small warning signals can be misunderstood by the brain to indicate that the injury is ongoing, where in fact the area is completely healed. Warning signals like this help to push the body towards the *Alert!* states and out of *Rest and Digest.*

Spreading pains

Pain from damage can easily spread from one side and then appear on the other side of the body too. A pain from a shoulder injury might spread to the other shoulder and into the top of the neck and upper back. This process is explained by the anatomy of where the nerves arrive in the brain, and it is possible for the messages to get muddled up. It does not mean there is additional damage in the body (or that the person is imagining it).

Spreading pain often indicates that there is a confusion in the brain, causing faulty signals. The faulty signals are processed as pain, so we feel pain where there isn't any damage. This process can happen to anyone and is not under our conscious control. It happens in all long-term physical pain conditions to some degree. This is called centralised pain. We can recognise centralised pain because one of its key features is that the pain seems to move about, or that it spreads from one area to another.

For instance, a single damaged joint will normally produce pain only around that joint. However, if the pain starts in one joint and then spreads to other places in the body, then the pain is becoming centralised. These spreading pains are evidence of the brain becoming confused and may indicate that brain inflammation is present.

This kind of pain is the one that is occurring in the fibromyalgia state, and in the next chapter we will explore how we can change it.

There is also growing evidence that our fascia (a type of connective tissue in the body) can create spreading pain. We will look at how fascia, acupuncture, and fibromyalgia are connected.

Surgery to try and cure pain

It is worth being aware that once pain from an injury has turned into a *centralised* pain, that doing surgery on that injury may not help to relieve all of the pain. Surgery can make any nerve damage worse in the area and may perpetuate the confusion. If you have a surgery planned, please discuss the outcomes for people with fibromyalgia with your surgeon[1].

If you think your condition just began with an injury and has now turned into chronic pain, I recommend you do all the same things suggested in the *Self-Help Tools* chapter (page 222). However the fibromyalgia state is initially triggered, the routes out again will be similar, as I will explain as we continue.

Be aware that elevated stress levels can exacerbate centralised pain, and even if you don't think stress was a cause of your condition, I recommend you do everything you can to give your body calming signals throughout the day that allow your brain chemistry to settle.

If you see a physical therapist, like an acupuncturist or masseuse, then do not ask them to treat all of the areas on your body that are painful. Instead ask them to only treat the original injury or (first) damaged area. Focus on the original injury and ask them to ignore the other pains. This should allow the brain to recalibrate better.

Acupuncturists who have taken a full training (3.5 year/degree level) will also know how to rebalance the autonomic nervous system, to help to calm the brain inflammation.

(A really brief) anatomy of acupuncture

Because my understanding of chronic pain is underpinned by my work as an acupuncturist, I want to give you a super brief anatomy of acupuncture to help explain a very important body part: the fascia.

Fascia is a type of connective tissue that allows our body to stretch a bit like elastic. It also allows different parts of the body to slide over or against each other. Under a microscope, it looks like layers of silvery threads like a mesh. Fascia has fibroblast cells that produce elastin and collagen (giving it a stretchy quality) and fasciacyte cells that produce hyaluran[2]. Hyaluran is a lubricant that allows our fascia to stretch smoothly and our tissues to glide over each other. (It is used in cosmetics to improve skin elasticity).

One of the reasons we know the fascia is involved in fibromyalgia is that there are changes in the concentration of hyaluran in fibromyalgia, as well as in other inflammatory diseases [34].

For decades, fascia was mistakenly thought to have no function in the body and it was typically thrown away during medical dissections. Only very recently, in the last twenty years, has research shown how amazing this elastic mesh in our body is.

Feeling our fascia

Fascia is the largest sensory organ in our body, larger in area than our skin! It has many more nerves in it than our muscles do, and fascia is around every one of our muscles.

If the fascia is not regularly moved, it can become matted. If this happens, it cannot transport fluids to the cells or slide properly as it should do. This matted effect can be seen under an electron microscope but cannot be seen using our usual health scanning techniques like ultrasound, x-ray, or MRI. Nervous tension and stress can also make the fascia contract, creating feelings of pain and stiffness.

Matted fascia feels achy or painful, but we can't feel it as distinctly different to muscles and so we tend to think the achy feeling is coming from the muscles. In the same way, we think we feel a headache is inside our brain, when actually there are no nerves inside our brain (we can actually only feel the outer layer of the brain.)

Fascia is interesting to acupuncturists because about 80% of all the acupuncture points, are located in the *fascia* [5] [6], often along lines of this connective tissue in the body that separate different body functions or muscle groups.

Acupuncture theory has always said that 'stagnation creates pain' and that areas of stagnation are often painful. We can now explain this idea from acupuncture with anatomical accuracy. Matted fascia is indeed a kind of stagnation and it creates pain, both widespread pains and in specific areas if there is damage there. The fact that acupuncture points are directed towards the fascia makes sense of acupuncture's ability to resolve pain in the body.

Fibromyalgia is very likely to have elements of matted fascia[7] because fibromyalgia pain is similar to the pain of fascia pain, and most people with fibromyalgia are not moving very much due to pain and fatigue.

Exercise has been shown to help with fibromyalgia but often it creates more soreness. So, with fibromyalgia, we need to make sure that the *type* of exercise we do is useful for the fascia. Performing exercise that just focuses on muscles is not helpful and may simply create more fatigue. On my website I can show you some simple fascia movements that you can try, see www.takingcontrol-fibromyalgia.co.uk. You can also read about Yin Yoga in the book, *From Fibromyalgia to Freedom* which I co-authored with two other therapists.

Fascia and nerve pain

If you've ever wondered why so much fibromyalgia pain can be felt in the skin, here is one explanation: the nerve endings near the very surface of our skin work in collaboration with special types of glial cells called *Schwann cells.*

Schwann cells have multiple 'filament connections' to the other surrounding glia cells in the skin[8] (they look at bit like an octopus with tentacles). They allow signals to travel *across* the skin surface between the cells, as well as along the nerves up to the brain, and they form a sensitive mesh of connected cells in the surface of the skin[9]. Schwann cells act as a surveillance system, reporting back to the brain about any injury near the skin surface, and they respond particularly to glutamate, signalling its presence[10].

Schwann cells have been seen to be expanded or 'ballooned' in people with fibromyalgia[11]. These cells sit in the fascia and our nerves should freely slide in the fascia as the body moves[12]. However, if the fascia tissue is matted or lacks hydration these nerves can be trapped or pulled. If the fascia is not allowing smooth movement then the tiny nerve endings can become slightly irritated. This mechanism has been proposed as the source of pain conditions that lack a visible cause[13].

5

HELPING OUR AUTONOMIC NERVOUS SYSTEM

A whole-body approach

As we have seen, our body is using glutamate for thinking, as well as a warning signal throughout the body, and so attempting to adjust the levels of glutamate in the brain with drugs is only ever going to be a short-term fix.

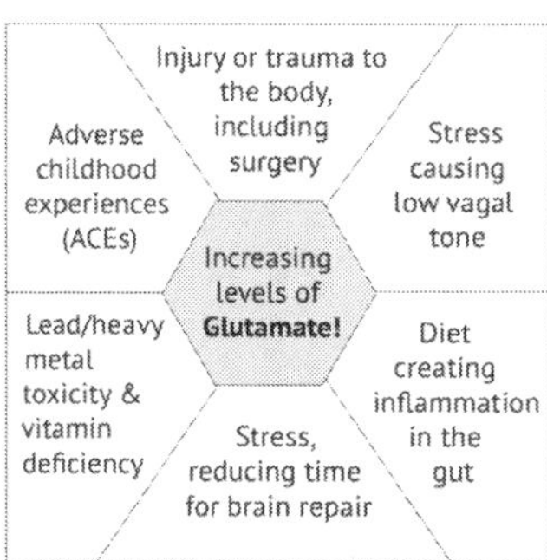

To regulate our glutamate levels for the long term, we need to balance the whole body, especially our nervous system, which carries warning signals from the body to the brain.

The time of our lives

Sometimes we are not aware of how stressed our body is. We get used to rushing about and being very busy and might not be in the habit of checking in with our internal feelings.

Stress is not a new problem. Humans have always been stressed; by our basic survival, by disease, by injury, and by other humans. However, the way we think about our lives has changed and we now expect our bodies to cope with things we regard as socially 'normal'.

Lighting is one example of something we all take for granted. However, it is only fairly recently, in the last century, that people in western Europe have had access to light whenever they want it. This one social change allows us to ignore the chronicity of daylight hours and work whenever we want. It also allows us to stay indoors to work, which hugely reduces our exposure to natural light.

Natural light is actually very important to our brains. Keeping away from blue light in the evenings is helpful and, in the mornings, a lightbox is a very useful tool. Small portable ones (about the size of an iPad) are available. Using one of these for a few hours in the mornings helps to reset the body clock and can help with both sleep rhythms and eye function. To avoid blue light in the evenings you can use filtering glasses or download apps to change screen colours, or even avoid all screens (phones, tablets and computers) in the evenings.

If I asked you to list stressful things in your life, lighting might not be top of the list, it might not even get onto the list, but for your body it might be having a bigger effect than you realise.

Letting our guts do the talking

We've seen that information goes directly from the gut to the brain. This means that looking after our body is very important for our brains.

If the brain receives constant warning signals about something being wrong in the body, it has an effect on the brain chemistry.

If our gut is not feeling good, due to inflammation or poor diet, the vagus nerve will carry the signals to our brain to say that there is a problem. What isn't so obvious is that our brain might experience those warning signals as 'indigestion' but it may also experience them as pain, depression, or even as anxiety! Long term, low levels of inflammation in the gut can have detrimental effects on the brain.

In fact, some psychiatrists are now proposing that our current treatment for depression, using drugs, is flawed. Instead, new models of depression suggest that we should be looking at the health of the entire body, and especially at inflammation, because of the effect of inflammation on the brain. Inflammation can cause the whole person to become depressed and withdrawn[1].

Irritable bowel syndrome (IBS)

Irritable bowel syndrome (IBS) is a kind of sensitivity that comes from a centralised brain effect, just like fibromyalgia. It is a condition that often shows up first, before fibromyalgia might start. IBS indicates that a problem between the gut and the brain is developing, like a low level of inflammation, or that gut permeability is increasing due to stress.

IBS is often food-related, but it is also very connected to stress. The gut and the brain are directly linked to each other by the vagus nerve; it is really important for the gut to tell the brain how it is feeling, so that the brain can do something about it. If we didn't have this connection the body would have no idea if something was good to eat again, or not.

Diets that reduce inflammation can make a big difference to fibromyalgia symptoms and I will outline some broad ideas about nutrition for fibromyalgia later on in this book.

You can also read detailed information about nutrition and

fibromyalgia in my co-authored book *From Fibromyalgia To Freedom.*

Diet as our safety net

The food we eat can directly influence our brain chemistry. The way we eat and at what times we eat, can also have an effect.

IBS indicates an early warning that we could be at risk of developing other inflammatory conditions. When we remember what the vagus nerve does, we can see how diet can contribute to a centralised pain condition like fibromyalgia, because the vagus nerve is carrying warning signals from the gut directly to the brain. However, this also works in our favour because it offers us a simple way to make changes to our brain.

The one idea it is useful to take away from this information is that because the gut and the brain are very closely linked, we can use what we eat, and the way we eat it, to tell our bodies that 'everything is ok'.

This is a cheap and easy way to actually change our body's response to stress!

Stress boils down to the body not feeling safe or not feeling comfortable. To counteract the effects of a stressful life we need to make the body feel safe and comfortable, and mostly this is an inside job. We need to be calm and comfortable INSIDE, rather than looking for a new sofa for our outsides!

Even if we cannot reduce the stress in our lives right now, we *can* help our body deal with it better.

Concluding this section....

In these chapters we have learnt that:

- Our autonomic nervous system controls the state we are in, in response to our environment.
- The vagus nerve has two parts, with different jobs (actions).
- Trauma can cause the autonomic nervous system to get stuck, either in a fearful and mobilised (ready to run) state, or in a *Shut-Down,* surrender state.

Later we will look at how to move out of fearful states and into *Rest and Digest.*

We also saw how the vagus nerve directly connects the gut and the brain:

- The gut tells the brain how it feels – through the vagus nerve.
- The autonomic nervous system can slow down our digestion, re-direct blood supply away from the gut, and towards the muscles instead.
- IBS can be an early indicator on a path towards fibromyalgia.
- Diet can be used as a tool to calm the brain.

What's next?

So far, we have looked at glutamate and chemistry, and at how our nervous system processes different kinds of stress, but what can we do about all the pain that occurs with fibromyalgia?

In the next section we are going to leave chemistry behind and explore centralised pain. How centralised pain can be caused, and how our mind interacts with pain.

PAIN

6

A PAIN THAT I'M USED TO

In spite of the enduring belief that the causes of fibromyalgia are all unexplained, there is actually lots of scientific research showing how fibromyalgia pain is caused.

You may be pleased to find out that although centralised pain can be called 'brain pain' it is definitely *not* 'all in your mind'.

A strange sting in the tail

I want to share with you a brief story about pain research to illustrate a common connection between painful events, chronic pain, and glutamate.

To research how pain can occur in the body, and to find pain-relieving medications to get rid of it, isn't very easy. Scientists generally have to start by creating some pain in a research animal, usually a rat. It is an unfortunate problem that animals are mainly used to research pain.

One way to induce a temporary pain is to inject a 1% acidic saline into a leg muscle. This is mildly painful but does not cause any actual damage to the muscle tissues themselves. The pain then wears off as the saline is absorbed naturally by the body.

I am telling you this because an unusual biological mechanism is triggered if the rat is given two injections in the same muscle, a few days apart. This *shouldn't* cause anything out of the ordinary to happen, as the rat is always well acclimatised to the procedures and lightly anaesthetised, so he should not be anticipating anything or be fearful. When the first injection is given, nothing 'unusual' happens in the rat, he just feels discomfort in that muscle.

However, when the animal is given a *second* injection, the researchers see that there is a release of glutamate both in the spinal cord and in the brain[1]. The rat then develops a heightened and long-lasting sensitivity to pain in other parts of his body. This is called muscle-induced hyperalgesia[2].

This effect can also be produced in humans by injecting extracts of chilli under the skin, or by stimulating the skin with electrical impulses so it becomes sore and sensitive.

What is hyperalgesia?

- Hyperalgesia means the body becomes *more* sensitive to pain.
- Hyperalgesia is a kind of neuropathic pain, which means it is caused by damage to the nervous system itself rather than being caused by damage to the body, (like in an injury to a muscle or a bone).
- Chemicals in the body can create hyperalgesia, but it can happen when there is no obvious physical cause.

Why would the rat's body respond this way? It doesn't seem logical to create a long lasting hypersensitivity to pain in response to a non-damaging injection.

However, the central nervous system appears to learn something from the first injection and when the second injection is administered the body responds in a stronger and maladaptive way.

Just like the immune system, the nervous system can 'learn' from previous events. We used to think that the nervous system and the immune system were quite separate, but they are now known to be working very closely together. The nervous system reacts differently to a second exposure of pain.

So, in the case of the rat who is being given a second injection, its nervous system is creating symptoms to get the body to move away from something that is perceived as dangerous.

Even tiny bacteria (most bacteria can move themselves) have a mechanism to move away from unhealthy chemicals (like alcohols) and towards useful things (like glucose). Moving the body away from sensory warning signals is hard-wired into our nervous system.

Muscle-induced hyperalgesia is a standard method used in laboratories to create a rat with chronic pain in order to test chronic pain medications and explore pain transmission pathways. For instance, if glutamate blocking drugs like ketamine are given to a rat with muscle-induced hyperalgesia, then the rat's pain goes away. Ketamine has a similar effect in humans too and it demonstrates that blocking glutamate receptors reduces this kind of pain. (Ketamine is, however, rarely used as a pain medication because it also causes nightmares, mood swings, hallucinations, and bladder problems.)

Causes of chronic pain sensitivity

This information from pain research shows how chronic pain can occur. If a healthy rat can develop chronic pain after having two non-damaging but painful injections, then we can see that a maladaptive (unhelpful) reaction to pain can be triggered in its body simply from experiencing a pain. This is similar to the way in which, in humans, surgery and injury can sometimes create long-lasting chronic pain or fibromyalgia.

Normally, an increased pain sensitivity like this will return to baseline levels and it will naturally go away. When it stays there, as we discussed in the previous chapter, then it is said to be a *centralised* problem. The brain and central nervous system are somehow continuing to produce the pain signals.

It is possible to produce centralised hyperalgesia in humans. This can be done experimentally using; electrical stimulation, capsaicin injections (chilli), mustard oil, acids, heat burns, UV burns, or with very salty injections (hypertonic saline)[3].

We know how to create increased pain sensitivity in a person, even without creating any damage to their body. As this is commonly known in pain science, I can't help wondering why so many doctors are claiming that fibromyalgia isn't a real condition.

While we are exploring hyperalgesia, we can take a short detour to discover how opioid drugs can *also* cause hyperalgesia.

Opioid drugs and fibromyalgia

Although opioid drugs are not recommended for fibromyalgia, you might be surprised to hear that they are still prescribed to sufferers. You may have heard about high doses of opioid drugs, or the long-term use of opioid drugs, making pain *worse* not better. This is because opioids also cause hyperalgesia.

This sounds slightly confusing, because opioids are supposed to be pain *killers*. For short-term use this is probably true, but if we keep taking them they have other effects.

We know that opioid hyperalgesia is caused by several mechanisms[4]:

- Opioid drugs inhibit our glutamate transport and recycling systems, allowing glutamate levels to *increase*.
- Long use of opioid drugs will kill some of our brain cells (neurotoxicity).
- Changes occur to the cells of the spinal cord in response to opioids, altering the cell receptors and moving the brain's chemistry away from 'normal' levels.
- Morphine can activate *astrocyte* and *microglia* cells (which should be in a 'resting' state) and these cells then produce inflammatory chemicals such as cytokines.

The other way that opioids can cause a problem is if the person's body is already making plenty of its *own* opioid pain killers. This is especially important information for fibromyalgia sufferers because it can set up a pattern known as latent sensitisation[5].

Latent sensitisation

Imagine someone called Mia cuts her hand badly. She has some stitches at the hospital but experiences quite a lot of pain from her hand.

Fortunately, her body has its own pain-reducing mechanisms and will produce its own natural pain-reducing chemicals in response to the pain. This natural pain-reducing mechanism includes the opioid receptors on her spinal nerve cells. [Our bodies use this system to help us cope with injury, childbirth, or any other painful event.]

After about a month, the pain in Mia's hand has pretty much gone and she feels fine.

Sometime after this, however, Mia experiences a lot of stress. She unexpectedly loses her job and has to look for a new one. During this period of stress, the pain in her hand comes back again. Mia doesn't understand why it hurts again, as it seemed to be completely healed.

Take your pain away

When Mia's hand stopped hurting, this was because her body was able to activate its own natural opioid receptors. This was all totally normal; her body was successfully dealing with any pain she experienced while her hand was healing.

However, her body might have *continued* to use her body's opioid receptors after the initial injury healed. For instance, in response to some lingering minor nerve damage in her hand. Again, this wasn't a problem and her body was coping well with the ongoing injury.

However, when Mia became stressed, the stress chemicals in her system increased. This mixture of stress chemicals, coupled with her natural opioid receptor activation, produced an unhealthy cocktail that was capable of tipping her central nervous system into a chaotic chemical state. Her nervous system had too many things to deal with and her brain was overloaded with warning signals.

This kind of chemical chaos can start to actually kill some brain cells, creating neuro-inflammation, and the brain becomes oversensitive to any incoming sensory messages.

In Mia's case, the minor nerve damage in her hand was no longer taken care of by her natural systems and instead this very minor damage started to cause her a lot of pain.

This is now a centralised pain, and the way that Mia's hand pain came back when she was stressed is called latent sensitisation.

This pattern, of a pain that goes away and then comes back during stress, can cause many chronic pain conditions. It can also cause problems when people are prescribed opioids. Old pains returning like this can create anxiety, and it is helpful to understand the biological mechanisms that allow it to happen.

Research: latent sensitisation is a fairly new model. It has been shown many times in rodents but there are not very many human studies yet. In 2013 one study was done in Copenhagen University Hospital (published in 2015). In this study, researchers created first-degree burns on the legs of twelve male volunteers, about the size of the palm of a hand. The men were tested daily on other parts of their body to see if they were developing increased pain sensitivity in *un*-injured areas.

After seven days they were given a drug that blocked all of their natural opioid receptors (naloxone). When the researchers did this, a quarter of the participants had significant changes to their pain levels. Four of the men felt *more* pain in un-injured areas as well as in the burn sites. This un-masking of hyperalgesia pain (increased pain sensitivity), shows that their opioid receptors were previously responsible for dealing with their burn pain.

The study was not very large, but it proved that latent sensitisation does occur in humans, as well as rats.

Opioids are not the cure

Returning to Mia's pain story: during the stressful time, when she is looking for a new job, Mia goes back to her doctor to ask for something for the hand pain that had returned.

If her doctor recognises that her pain is a hyperalgesia caused by latent sensitisation, he may recommend calming activities or education. But it's possible that her doctor doesn't know about latent sensitisation, and instead gives her an opioid painkiller.

Mia takes the drugs and this *prescribed* opioid circulates around her body, but all the opioid attachment sites on the nerve cells are *already activated* by Mia's own natural pain-reducing mechanisms.

This means that Mia doesn't get much pain relief from the prescribed opioid drugs. All the prescribed ones can do is to add to the chemical cocktail washing around her nerves, creating drug side effects like drowsiness. If Mia increases her dose, thinking that it will help, then her chemistry just gets further out of balance.

People with fibromyalgia have increased levels of their own natural opioids, and they have reduced numbers of opioid receptor sites on their cells[6]. This is the reason that opioids are not recommended for fibromyalgia, and probably why opioids have not shown to have any good effects on fibromyalgia pain.

It is worth noting that hyperalgesia (increased pain sensitivity) caused by drugs is not the same as 'tolerance'. Tolerance to a drug can be overcome by increasing the dose but hyperalgesia gets *worse* if the dose is raised.

Need to know

Prescribed opioid drugs are more likely to work in the initial stages of an injury, and only for about a week. If people keep taking opioids for ongoing pain then their system can end up becoming more and more sensitised. Their pain gets worse, not better.

This is why opioids are not recommended for fibromyalgia.

The fibromyalgia and chronic pain specialist at the University of Michigan, Dr. Clauw, says that using opioids for fibromyalgia is like trying to put out a fire by adding petrol to it.

If you are taking opioids for fibromyalgia, you should consult your doctor to make a plan so that you can wean yourself off these medications gradually.

Fortunately, research shows that the hyperalgesia caused by opioid drugs only lasts for about a month[7].

Placebo… or is it the real one?

What is fascinating about latent sensitisation is that it ties up with what a 'placebo' is. We have all been schooled to think of a placebo as a fake thing (like a sugar pill instead of a drug) that works on *some* people. There has been a tendency to think that people who respond to a placebo are more gullible or easily suggestible. That was until we found out where placebo actions actually take place in the body.

The effects of placebos take place in those same opioid receptors[8], the ones that helped Mia to reduce her pain naturally. People who respond to placebos are the ones whose bodies have a really good and effective mechanism to deal with pain. Their own inbuilt pain system works well. That's probably why they are so easily triggered by swallowing a sugar pill, or something similar – because it doesn't take much to switch their own system on.

It is possible to do brain scans and see which people will respond well to placebos, because this has to do with the way the brain is wired and connected. Rather than being weak-minded or hysterical, the people who respond well to placebos are actually the ones who score highly for resiliency, altruism (generosity), and straightforwardness, and low on measures of 'angry hostility'.[9]

Having *lower* cortisol levels also helps placebos to work better. Cortisol is a stress hormone and high levels are an indicator of too much stress. So, lowering stress levels helps our natural pain management system work more easily. One thing that stops placebos from working is fear. Expecting bad things to happen is simply instructing our brain to be on alert and look for 'bad things', whereas being hopeful or optimistic is a calmer outlook on life.

Placebo responders are not unusual. 33% of us are responsive to placebo-induced pain relief[10], which indicates that a natural non-drug mechanism for pain relief is present in all of us, and that for some people their pain reduction system is very easy to switch on.

The part of the brain that controls our natural system of pain management is called the periaqueductal grey (PAG) and this can be activated by acupuncture, which helps to explain acupuncture's ability to treat pain[11].

It's possible that many medical drugs may actually diminish or block our natural pain-reducing effects[12], in the same way that opioid drugs have been seen to do. Hopefully in the future we will all be working to maximise our natural systems, and this is a large part of what I want to encourage you to do in order to treat your fibromyalgia.

In this chapter, we have learned that:

- Repeated pain experiences can make the body more sensitive to pain.
- Increased pain sensitivity is called hyperalgesia.
- If increased pain sensitivity continues, then it is assumed to

be caused by the brain and spinal cord (the central nervous system) and is then called *centralised pain.*

- Opioids are not recommended for fibromyalgia and can make chronic pain worse[13].
- Opioid drugs include tramadol, co-codamol, codiene, oxycodone, fentanyl, buprenorphine, hydrocodone, and methadone.
- The 'placebo' effect is just a natural pain-reducing mechanism that is present in all of us.
- It is likely that fibromyalgia has several causes and that more than one trigger is required in order to create it in the body.

So, in the following chapters we will find other parts of this fibromyalgia jigsaw, and then we can look at ways in which we might be able to reverse these processes.

7

EVERYBODY HURTS

We might ask: how do we feel pain?

We know pain is a warning that we have hurt ourselves, and so we might imagine that pain is something that happens, and then the nervous system sends '*pain*' signals to the brain, but this is not actually the case.

Pain is actually the *result* of lots of different kinds of signals that come to the brain from the nervous system. Our brains create pain, from all of the signals they receive.

The brain has the ability to collect available information, to interpret and 'understand' it. There are sensory nerves in many places such as our skin, muscles, and fascia. These 'peripheral' nerves (coming from the *periphery*, furthest from the brain) send signals about the body, along the nerves, to the spinal cord and the brain. These are the journalists from our body-organisation analogy.

These signals from the body can be simple 'check-in' signals, or they can be warning signals. Pain is produced as an *interpretation* of these signals. The brain looks at all the evidence it has and decides if something should be painful.

Your brain is just managing

If there is a report of a mechanical sensation coming from the nerve endings in your skin, the nervous system sends these signals to your brain, and your brain might decide that something is touching your neck. The brain will use other information to decide how it wants your body to react to this touch. The brain also uses auditory input (sound), sight, and memories to inform its decisions.

It might decide that the thing touching you is just a label in your clothing and that no action is required. Alternatively, it might remember that you were once stung by an insect in your clothing and send signals to immediately search for the source of that touch!

We'd like to think that our brains work like computers, analysing information carefully and rationally, but it isn't really quite like that.

I know I said earlier that the brain is like a managing director, but I didn't tell you very much about that managing director. Instead of a calm and rational managing director (MD), imagine instead that your brain is more like a rather nervous person who accidentally found themselves in charge of this huge organisation, and who hasn't really got a clue how to run it.

This nervous MD might decide, if there is too much information being thrown at them, to just run away and hide in a cupboard for a while. They can get confused by things, and mostly they just want everything to be ok so that they can concentrate on finding a nice place to eat dinner.

For clarity, I'm going to continue to call the physical lump of grey stuff in your skull 'the brain' and refer to *you*, the thinking personality that I am speaking to, as 'the mind'.

[I'm also going to make our brain MD male, because it's easier, and most MDs – whether we like it or not – still are male.]

Why does the brain create pain?

The body and brain have to communicate with each other. In order to keep us safe the brain takes all the information it has and tries to keep us away from things that are dangerous. If the brain remembers fear, or if it receives sensory information that it thinks is a warning, then it may want the body to move away from these signals. Pain can be one way the brain can get the body to move away from something dangerous, like a hot stove.

There is a lot of research evidence that *sensory information*, something you can feel (like your skin being pinched), is not enough to cause pain on its own. The brain has to interpret the pinching as a threat, and only then are pain signals created to get you to move out of the way [1] [2].

So, if the brain receives a report about a touch sensation like a very light breeze, and the ears hear a rumbling sound, and the eyes see a light approaching, and the memory says '*you should stand back from a train line*', we may suddenly jump away in fear just from the feeling of a light breeze!

All sensory information (called *nociception* in science) has to go through the brain before the brain decides whether it is a threat or not, and in this example it decided that the feeling of a light breeze – combined with what it saw and heard – indicated a danger that we needed to move away from, fast!

Pain is also not created in relation to how much damage the body has. Even though, in our normal experience, we tend to believe that *more damage = more pain,* most of us actually have lots of structural damage. Many people have damage present in their spine for instance (which can be seen on scans), but experience no pain at all from any of it[3].

For instance, by twenty years old 37% of people have disc degeneration and 30% have a disc bulge. Most twenty-year-olds do not have back pain and plenty of people over fifty are also pain free. This shows us that pain might be caused by damage, but not all damage causes pain.

Kind of damage	20 years old	40 years old	50 years old
Disc degeneration	37%	68%	80%
Disc bulge	30%	50%	60%

Pain does not always mean there is damage – it means that the brain is worried that the signals it is receiving are dangerous.

Stress can create similar effects to injuries

The central nervous system has similar responses to a lot of different warning signals. We can see this in action if we look at two examples: firstly, the way the central nervous system responds to body damage, and then how it responds to a stressful event.

1) Body damage

If the body is damaged in some way, for instance in an accident or from surgery, then acute inflammation is caused by the tissue damage. This inflammation activates the autonomic nervous system, which switches the body into the mobilised and fearful states – *Alert!, Fright, Flight or Fight* – and releases adrenaline.

Due to this inflammation, more glutamate is released and the levels of glutamate increase.

The brain processes all these warning signals, along with memories and other information (like seeing the damage to the body) and produces pain signals to stop us from moving that part, so that it can heal.

2) Stress effects

When our stress levels increase, the autonomic nervous system moves the body into the fearful and mobilised states – *Alert!, Fright, Flight or Fight*. Switching into these fearful or mobilised states can in itself increase our glutamate levels.

Glutamate is an inflammatory chemical that at high levels can kill neurons, creating more inflammation and more warning signals in the brain. Inflammation and high glutamate levels can create pain sensitivity and amplify sensory signals.

You can see how these two things, damage and stress, have very similar chemical effects and how, if both are occurring at once, the brain might begin to get pretty muddled up about what is actually going on in the body.

The body can easily start to regard stress as a damaging event, similar to an injury.

This is one way that the brain may learn and remember that stress is dangerous and start to increase the warning signals it creates when experiencing stress.

Response to damage leads to higher glutamate levels

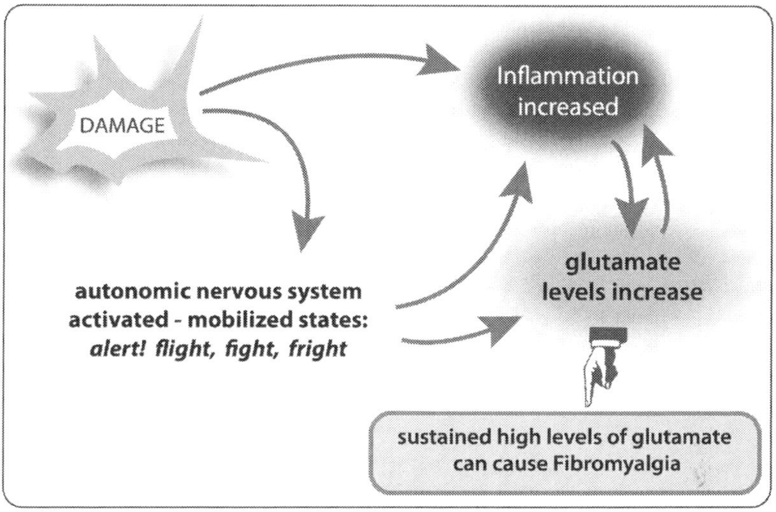

Possible effects of stress

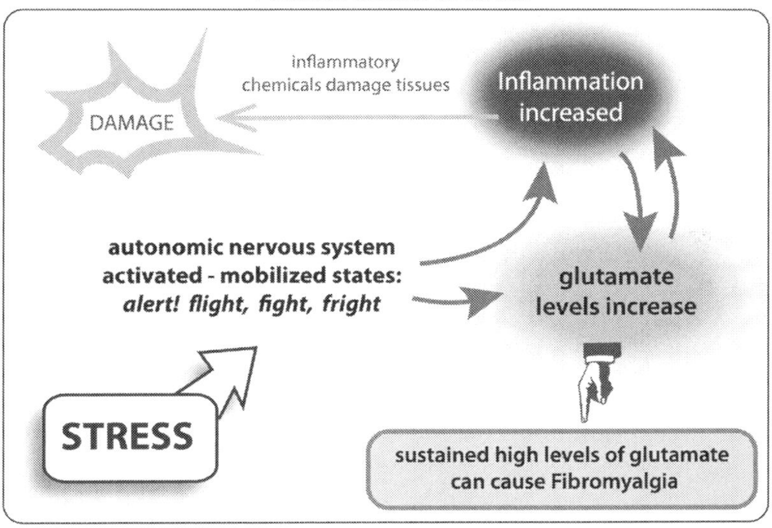

Pain and warnings

Pain is not a straightforward process of something going wrong and the brain being told about it. This is important because we tend to feel that all pain means something is wrong or broken in our body. As we have seen, however, damage is not always the reason that pain occurs.

The relationship between 'threat' and 'pain' is very close. The brain is keeping watch in order to help us to avoid situations it remembers as being dangerous or stressful.

Fear is an anticipation of something that might happen, and fear is well known to create more pain than when fear is not present. Fear increases pain. Both fear and pain are feelings that are created to keep us away from things that are bad for us.

Knowing that pain does not indicate that something is broken is very useful to us, and we can reassure ourselves we are ok. Lots of kinds of pain, from stabbing pains to aches, and pins and needles or headaches, can be feelings created by the brain when the brain gets muddled. Chronic pains are just another warning signal and they often exist without any actual damage at all.

Pain can change

In my own practice I have got rid of long standing, chronic pains for many people. Sometimes the pain has resolved very quickly and my client is amazed that somehow I have, for instance, 'fixed' their back. Sometimes they have had a back pain for many years. They had assumed that since no-one could get rid of the pain for them before, then they must have extensive damage to their spine. Sometimes they have had scans showing areas of damage that seem to confirm this.

In reality, the faster people get better, the more likely it is that there was no damage left at all, and the brain was simply continuing to create pain. The acupuncture helped with this brain pain and it simply went away, even though the scans may show no change has occurred. For years, some people thought acupuncture might be a kind of sophisticated placebo. Today, if we use the definition of placebo that I gave you earlier, we can say: yes, it is, and it works on many people to help their brain to reduce pain.

We are designed to cope with lots of damage; the human body is an amazing, creative and flexible organism.

Our brain is just trying to work out what is dangerous and what is ok. It creates pain in order to keep us safe. Adding fear or stress to sensory signals is likely to convince the brain that there is danger and it is then more likely to produce pain.

We know that fear and stress change our brain chemistry (via the autonomic nervous system) making pain more likely or more intense.

Pain theories

There are two main theories about how pain is created, and these ideas lead us in two different directions to find treatments for pain. If we take a look at these two ideas, we'll see why they suggest different options for reducing pain.

The first idea about pain is the most commonly used one, called central sensitisation.

Most studies on chronic pain regard the central nervous system as being 'over-sensitised'. This is the chemical model that we explored in our first chapters. We can measure that there is too much glutamate in the brain and spinal cord, and this leads to multiple bio-chemical processes being out of balance.

This idea says that sensory inputs from the nerves go up to the brain correctly, but in the brain they are all muddled up, because the brain is being oversensitive. The neurons start to trigger each other without being told to and cause a 'wind-up', like feedback loops in the system.

In our body organisation, the sensory journalists are sending all the reports up to the MD as usual, but his desk is a mess. Plus, he's been taking a load of chemicals, either stress chemicals from the journalists, or maybe inflammation chemicals from the gut, and he's feeling a bit overwhelmed. Consequently, he's not dealing with the work very well and is complaining that it just all hurts.

Medical treatments based on the idea of central sensitization use drugs to try to rebalance brain chemicals. Drugs are used to block receptor sites in the nerve cells in the brain, so that the brain calms down. These treatments have some success but changing the way the brain chemicals work tends to also create unwanted side effects for the person taking the drugs.

Other ideas

The second idea is newer and is not so well known.

Another way to understand what is going on in chronic pain is the imprecision hypothesis of chronic pain (I'm sorry none of these ideas have very catchy names!)

This idea says that the brain is not oversensitive; it is doing its job correctly, however it has forgotten which signals are dangerous and which ones are safe. It is interpreting *all* body signal as dangerous and therefore makes everything feel painful. This kind of brain confusion would mean that the brain starts paying attention to really minor signals and deals with them as if they serious emergencies. Lots of warning signals are produced in the brain and this leads to the imbalance of the brain chemistry.

In the body organisation, lots of our routine signals that go from the body to the MD and the board of directors (the central nervous system) are normally filtered, so that the MD only has to think about some of them. But in this situation, it's like the MD has been up all night watching horror films. Now he's at work he's got really himself really worried and paranoid and has decided that he needs to personally listen to every single incoming report.

He has turned up the volume in his office so that all of the reports are really loud and he doesn't miss anything, which also makes them sound much more scary than they actually are. He's working hard to get all of these reports checked, but he's in a bit of a panic and is issuing warnings and pain signals all over the place. He's sending out instructions saying that every report could be a really scary potential problem.

This theory points us towards treatments that help the body and brain to relearn which things are safe and which are not. This kind of learning is done using the body itself in order to affect the mind. We can use specific movements and stress-relieving treatments that affect the nervous system, to teach the brain that not everything is dangerous.

To make the treatment options clear for us, we can also use Pavlov's dog to demonstrate the differences for us.

Pavlov's dog

You may have heard about how Dr. Pavlov's dog reacted to a training programme.

Dr. Pavlov rang a bell before he gave his dog some food and after a while of doing this, the dog started to salivate (drool) only from the sound of the bell ringing, before Dr. Pavlov produced any dog food.

This is called a conditioned response, a learned behaviour, one that can be triggered by something that is unrelated to the result. (In this case, just a sound, not the food itself). This is normal, healthy, brain behaviour.

This kind of learning helps us to anticipate things in the world. The dog's brain learned that the sound of the bell means food is coming. After a while, the nervous system of the dog produced saliva just when it heard the bell.

Dr. Pavlov's dog can also demonstrate our pain theories for us.

Let's imagine Pavlov had three dogs, and they responded differently to the training:

The first dog was carefully trained, and he behaved as he was expected to, as described above. At the end of his training the bell was rung, and the dog started to salivate.

The second dog behaves differently. He demonstrates the central sensitisation theory; after his training, when the bell is rung, this dog does lots of other behaviours, things other than just salivating. He sits down, runs around, jumps up, or barks.

You could imagine that this second dog gets over-excited when he hears the bell and his responses get all muddled up.

Pavlov's third dog demonstrates the imprecision hypothesis. This time, the bell was rung and the dog salivated correctly, but this dog *also* salivates if the door slams, if the lights are turned on, if a car passes outside, or if Dr. Pavlov sneezes.

Here, the *stimulus* is muddled up. This third dog responds correctly, but he responds to lots of different kinds of sound. The dog's brain interprets many random events as a cue to salivate.

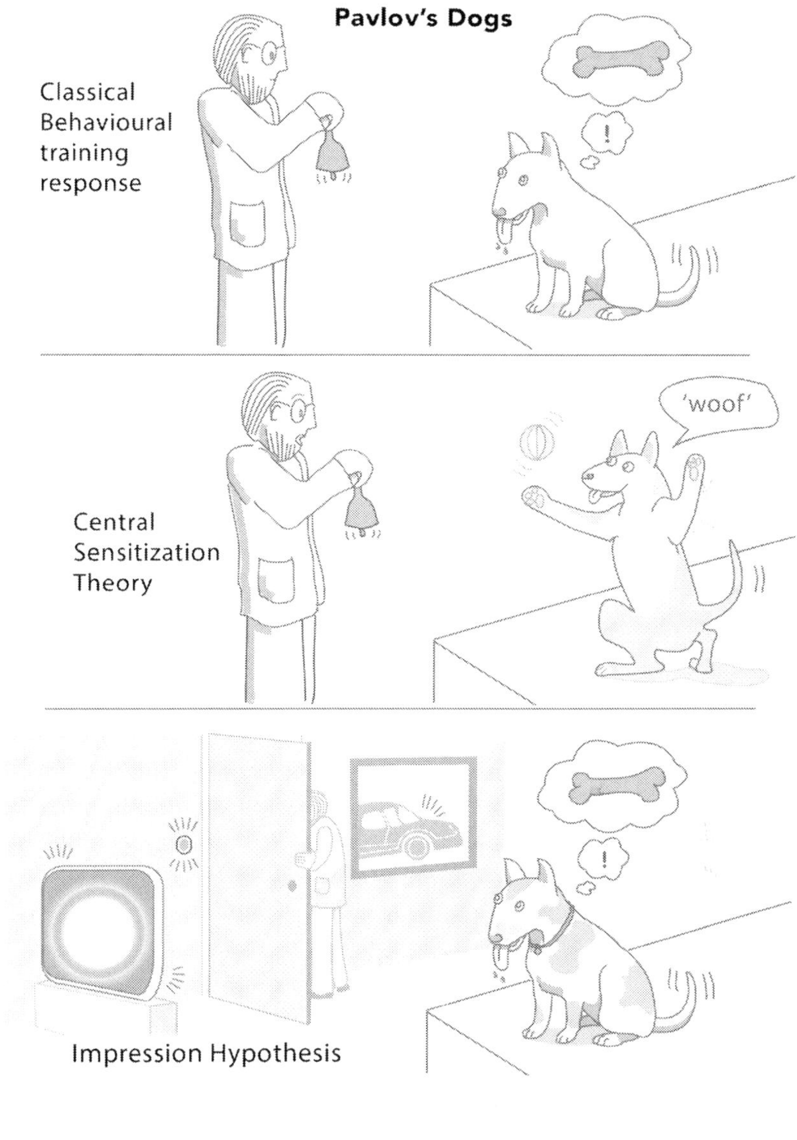

Applying these ideas to fibromyalgia

Imagine that Dr. Pavlov's wife strained a muscle in her back and that for the first few days it only hurt if she turned sideways to the left.

However, the following month the pain is all over her back, and it hurts if she bends her back only a little way. She also has a stiff neck, arm pains, and some headaches too. This pain continues and does not get better over the coming months. She has the choice to see two different doctors:

A doctor using the central sensitisation theory might diagnose Mrs. Pavlov as having a chronic hyperalgesia (pain sensitivity). He would say that her brain and central nervous system are acting incorrectly and that her brain chemicals are out of balance.

This doctor would give her drugs, like pregabalin, to regulate her brain chemicals.

However, if Mrs. Pavlov wanted a second opinion, she might go to a doctor who uses the imprecision hypothesis. This doctor would say that Mrs. Pavlov's brain is doing the correct thing, but that her brain has decided the original muscle injury was very dangerous. Her brain is now on alert and signalling to the brain that *every* movement is dangerous. The body is over-protecting her by stopping her from moving much at all.

This doctor might give her very slow and gentle exercises to do, with some mind training and acupressure, to reprogramme the brain's interpretation of movement.

The self-help tools in this book use this second theory – the imprecision hypothesis of pain because it helps us to find all-natural solutions to pain. The scientists who developed the theory describe it as 'brain pain', which is easier to remember (and type) than the imprecision hypothesis of pain.

Although the biochemistry of central sensitisation is useful information for us, the treatments created by it are just more drugs. However, drugs are not very effective for treating chronic pain, and they also cause many unwanted side effects.

In this book I will show you how you can use body-based therapies to change and resolve the 'brain pain' to resolve fibromyalgia.

Pain Theories to understand Fibromyalgia

Central sensitization	Imprecision Hypothesis
What does the theory say?	
Brain makes extreme or disordered responses to normal body signals	Brain makes makes normal pain responses ...but responds to the wrong signals (neutral signals)
Evidence	
Brain chemicals are changed i.e. higher levels of glutamate	Heightened skin sensitivity (Hyperalgesia)
How does each theory help us?	
Understanding how brain chemistry can both create and maintain chronic pain conditions like fibromyalgia	Understanding how repeated pain can cause pain sensitivity (hyperalgesia). The brain 'learns' incorrect connections and has blurry maps
What treatments does each theory indicate?	
Drugs like PCP, Pregabalin, Ketamine (but also therapies such as acupuncture and Yoga)	Body based therapies, like acupuncture, Yoga & Stress relieving activities like breathing and meditation

Pain as protection

We have seen that the body uses pain to stop us from doing things that are damaging to us. The pain scientist Professor Lorimer Moseley tells a story about working with an elite cyclist who had a back pain that only happened when the cyclist was cycling up hills. He was wondering if her pain was purely mechanical or if it was connected with her brain's interpretation of hills.

To test this idea, he put her on a static treadmill bike with a screen in front of it and then on the screen he showed her films so *it looked like* she was cycling up a hill. This immediately brought on the back pain. This demonstrated that the pain was created from unconscious memories of hills.

We could guess that maybe in the past the cyclist hurt herself or felt really sore after cycling up a hill once, or maybe on a few occasions. We don't know the frequency required, but her brain had connected *cycling-up-hills* with *damage*, so that when the brain saw the bike (apparently) going up a hill, it perceived a threat and activated pain signals to try and stop her from cycling up it.

Once the cyclist understood that her back pain was just a kind of cognitive association, and the pain was not related to any actual damage, she stopped having the pain. She stopped worrying about the feeling and the feeling went away.

At times, we can all be fooled by our brain. If we feel pain, we quite naturally assume that we are damaged somewhere, but this might not always be the case. New pain science is revealing that pain can be caused by damage we can see, and also from the chemistry in the brain. However, there is still confusion about what this means. One example of a confusion is the idea that stress is the *cause* of the pain, and that 'stress' is the patient's fault somehow. Stress can contribute to chronic pain, as we have seen, but in itself it is not a cause. So, in the next section we will get clear about what is going on.

Real or un-real pain

Is there a difference between types of pain? No. There isn't any difference, and this is particularly important in relation to chronic pain conditions like fibromyalgia. All pain is real. There is no difference at all between pain triggered by a damaged part of the body and pain that is created by the brain (the medical profession call this 'psychogenic' pain). They are *exactly the same pain*, just triggered from different causes, and they often occur together.

In any chronic pain condition, some of the pain is coming from brain chemistry. This means that all chronic pain conditions have an element of 'brain pain'. Fibromyalgia is believed to be almost all coming from brain chemistry, but even someone with arthritis pain, where we can see physical joint damage on their scans, has 'brain pain' too. It is not possible to say that one person has brain pain and another person doesn't; we now know that everyone with chronic pain has some degree of it.

An iceberg of pain

You may be wondering… if chronic pain is involved with the brain interpreting signals wrongly, or in a muddled way, are we aware of this happening? And are we responsible for these processes?

For the last twenty years I have worked with people experiencing many types of acute and chronic pain and I am always disappointed to hear that a medical professional has been dismissive or judgemental about a client's experience of pain. There are some incorrect myths about the creation of pain. So, I would like to address these from a psychological perspective, to answer these questions about awareness and responsibility.

All in the mind

What the phrase 'all in the mind' normally refers to is something *invented* in the conscious mind. This is *not* what happens in chronic pain. Yes, the *awareness* of pain is in the conscious mind. However, we can prove that pain learning, and pain responses, are learned and triggered by *un*conscious processes in the brain[4].

'Pain is experienced in our conscious mind, but created in our unconscious mind'[5].

Is it out of my control?

Not completely; we can still *influence* pain consciously, even when it is created unconsciously. For instance, conscious perception of 'how threatening something is' is known to influence our pain reactions.

This means we can use our conscious mind to reassure our nervous system.

Reducing our fear of pain is one method of doing this, which is why I wanted to share with you the information about how pain is created – because pain is just a warning signal and does not necessarily mean anything in the body is damaged, we can reassure ourselves that it is possible to be fine and be in pain at the same time.

An expectation of pain

Expectation makes any pain worse in humans (and rats too). How we remember and understand our environment alters the way our brain interprets things that happen to us.

For instance, in one experiment, two groups of people were given a small electrical stimulation to their skin. This electrical stimulation usually makes the skin a bit more sensitive to pressure tests for a short time afterwards.

One group were given instructions that said: 'After the electrical stimulation, your skin will become more sensitive to a pinprick test'. The other group did not receive this information. The group who were told to expect more sensitivity *did* experience more pain when they were tested.

This is why reassuring our self does work to help ease pain.

Pain psychology

I'm sharing ideas with you about how to take control of pain, which is me talking to the conscious part of you. I also said earlier that pain is *felt* consciously but *created* unconsciously. So, how do parts of the mind work together to create and resolve pain?

I want to be very clear about the parts of our mind in relation to pain.

For too long, there have been some pretty awful assumptions about patients being responsible for creating their own pain or about repressed feelings being converted into pain.

Feelings and thoughts have a direct effect on pain, but that does not mean that feelings and thoughts *create* pain.

[We know this because it has not been possible to create pain with a conditioned response training.]

Conscious or unconscious

The conscious and unconscious are often talked about, and often only these two, however there are actually three states of consciousness: the conscious, the *pre*conscious and the unconscious.

You might like to imagine your mind as being like parts of an iceberg. The top part you can see, that sticks up out of the water, is your conscious mind. There is another part just under the water which is the preconscious. As you go further down and there is less light, thoughts become invisible to you and this is the unconscious.

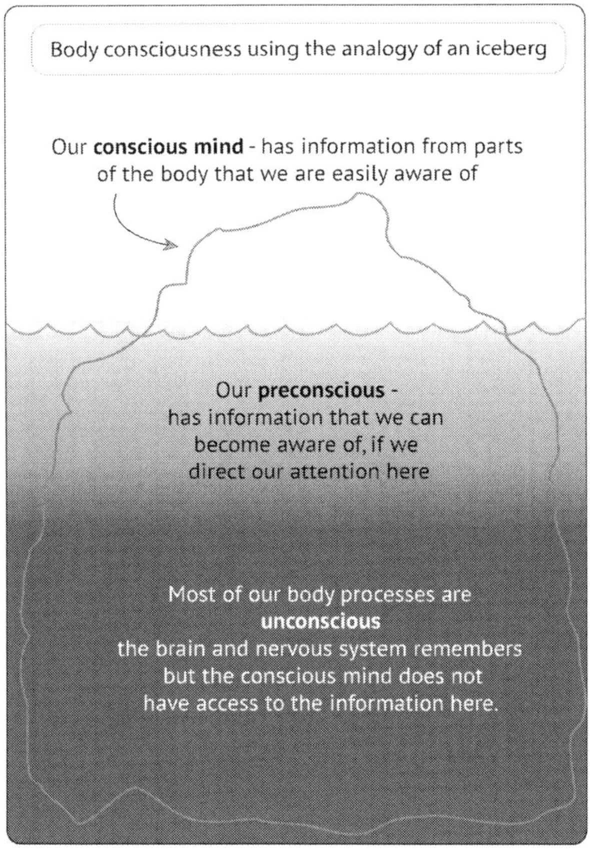

Parts of our mind

These three parts (or functions) of our mind each has a relationship with how we feel and experience things in the world.

We use our conscious mind to 'feel' pain.

This part of our mind has information we can easily be aware of. For instance, what we can touch, see, or hear around us, and maybe how we feel emotionally.

When we are under anaesthetic sedation, we feel no pain because our conscious mind is temporarily shut-down. This makes surgery much more acceptable.

The preconscious contains thoughts, feelings and memories that we are not aware of, until we look for them.

We can bring things from our preconscious into the conscious mind if we direct our attention there. For instance, in our body we might normally be unaware of our heartbeat, or our breathing, but when we look for this information we *can* feel and become aware of these body processes.

Our unconscious is the part of our mind and body that we cannot be aware of.

It includes things like the neural pathways in our brain and spinal cord. There are no sensory nerves inside our brain so we cannot 'feel' it. There is no method to bring this information into our conscious mind naturally. If someone touches our foot, we are aware of the touch but we are not aware of the route the signals took to get from our foot to our brain, or even where in our brain those signals were turned into an interpretation of touch. These things are unconscious processes.

Memories can be conscious, pre-conscious, or unconscious.

Sometimes, we can remember things easily, like where we live. This memory is available to your conscious mind.

Alternatively, we might have to think and concentrate to remember something, like where we left our keys. This is a pre-conscious memory.

And sometimes our unconscious mind remembers things, like an association or a smell. This can be information that our conscious mind does not know that we know.

Pain is partly based on memories. We probably have memories of things that were dangerous or have hurt us in the past, and about things only hurt for a short time and then we felt better. We might consciously remember these events or sometimes the unconscious may have just stored the memory for us in case we need it.

Memory helps the brain work better because there is less to decide today if we remember what happened last time. Mostly, this is useful but occasionally it's not.

The mind makes guesses

Every day when we wake up, our brain cannot start from scratch, working out how the world works. It would take too long and we would have to repeat loads of learning each day. Instead, the brain works using prediction.

It predicts that today, most of the world will be the same as it was yesterday.

I will, for instance, still be a human being and the physical world will behave as it did yesterday; gravity will be the same, trees don't talk, and I still won't like the taste of grapefruit. Instead of learning all these things over and over again, my brain remembers the world from previous days (and years). This way, it can concentrate on today and on learning new things, which is much more interesting and stops me from buying a grapefruit every day to see if I'll like it.

This prediction technique works *very well* to keep the conscious brain from being overwhelmed by too much information.

But it works *very badly* when we have pain, or depression, or any other ongoing unpleasant condition, because the brain just starts each day where it left off yesterday.

So, if there was chronic widespread pain yesterday, it predicts that there will be chronic widespread pain today. This becomes just another static piece of information in our memory… unless something changes.

The brain also makes predictions about tomorrow too, and it makes them based on today. So, if today felt like a bad day then it will predict that tomorrow is unlikely to feel really good, or that *any* day in the future could be better than this one.

These predictions can mean that some people actually give up hope that things are able to change, or do nothing to change their situation because it 'feels' like the future couldn't be very different to how it feels today.

[This prediction effect is called affective forecasting. The psychologist Daniel Gilbert wrote an excellent and entertaining book about it called '*Stumbling on Happiness.*']

Why is this important for fibromyalgia sufferers? Because as long as we know that the brain works like this, we can work with it to improve how we feel. We can *consciously* imagine a different future. We can *consciously* change things that help our brain to relearn a new set of 'norms', even if we have had pain for a very long time.

Memories, movement, and pain

It is common when we have experienced a physical pain for our bodies to start associating movement with pain, like the cyclist who had unconsciously associated hills with her back pain.

One idea about how pain and movement can become connected is that the brain collects signals and memories in little bundles called neurotags.

Neurotags

Neurotags are the name given to a group of connected signals in the brain.

For instance, we may have experienced ourselves that a memory can get attached to a pop song, or a memory might be connected to a certain location, or a feeling might be connected to a certain smell. These are associations in the brain between different things. And these connections can be created and strengthened by repetition, coincidence, or just by error (brain mistakes).

A neurotag could be a perception, a thought, a movement, or even an immune system response. We could think of a neurotag as a file with some information in it.

Groups of synapses (brain cells) are fired to produce a memory and because they have been connected previously, they have stronger connections between then. When one cell fires it also sets off its related cells.

I tend to imagine, in this instance, that our memory is like a library full of reports, and that those reports sit next to each other on shelves. (Please forgive me for this analogy if you have neuroscience training!).

It's pretty easy for information in the reports to get stuck to each other, especially if the reports are pulled out on a regular basis to be looked at.

If our memory librarian goes to get the report for a song we like and, every time they go to that shelf, they notice the nearby report is about a memory connected to that song, we might ask to see both files. If we keep opening both those files together the librarian might just file them together, to save time. Now that song and the memory are part of the same neurotag (file).

Neurotags can become 'blurred' at the edges, so that when one neurotag is triggered, nearby neurotags can be triggered too. Blurring of neurotags like this allows brain interpretations to get a bit muddled, like Dr. Pavlov's third dog.

Later, I'll show you some ways we can easily demonstrate this blurring effect.

Using neurotags to treat fibromyalgia

Movement can get connected to pain. Any movement can then start to trigger warnings in the brain, which creates pain to make us stay still. Staying still is ok for reptiles, but not it's not ok for humans!

Our bodies are designed to move, and things go wrong when we don't. Our tissues can become too acidic if we don't move, and our lymphatic system has to work hard to clean our tissues without movement. Both of these problems can create pain themselves, which is why so much research shows that moving about improves pain.

One thing we can do to counter the 'pain-connected-to-movement' effect, is to slowly do new or unusual movements.

Putting the body in unusual positions that feel safe and relaxed, can teach the brain to make new neural connections. It breaks the pattern, so that movement-and-pain are disconnected.

This doesn't mean you need to start doing tonnes of exercise; even simple slow things can be good. In the tools section I'm going to teach you to find acupressure points, which will mean you touching your skin in places to find the points. Even this simple movement will be new to your brain and could start to create new movement neurotags.

We need to be relaxed and feel safe in order for these new connections to be helpful. If we were stressed or anxious while moving, we would just add another new 'warning' signal to the neurotag for that movement.

Making *slow and deliberate* movements with gentle slow breathing can be especially helpful to undo unhelpful warning signals that have become attached to our movement neurotags. Slow types of yoga, like Yin Yoga, and some fascial release movements like *The Melt Method* are especially good for fibromyalgia.

Pain as a guard dog

Pain is a warning signal from the unconscious parts of our body to the conscious parts. It says: "Pay attention, something might be wrong!"

Sometimes the unconscious part of our mind remembers something from the past and it adds this information to things that are happening now.

This is why some pain professionals talk about pain being 'learned' pain. You, in your mind, did not do this learning but your unconscious might have, because 'pain' is created from a combination of sensory signals and from all kinds of memories.

Let's say you were running one day, and you were enjoying it, and your brain might have been using a LEG-RUNNING-FUN neurotag, where running and fun are connected. Then one day you fell and hurt your leg, and so your brain has a memory that your leg hurt, and it was painful when it was moved, so it created a new neurotag; LEG-MOVING-WARNING! This new neurotag is used to stop you moving that leg too much until it heals. Normally, once your leg was healed your brain would update the temporary LEG-MOVING-WARNING! neurotag back to LEG-RUNNING-FUN again.

However, if the body is dealing with lots of emergencies, like stress, inflammation, being on high-alert, or has multiple areas of damage, then the neurotags don't get updated correctly. Things start to get into a muddle.

We are hard-wired to respond to pain and to avoid it. All animals limp if they hurt their feet or legs, no-one teaches them to do this.

This avoidance of pain is completely normal, so it might feel rather unusual if I suggest that you say to your body: "Okay, I'm going to proceed as if this pain is a false alarm. My body's guard dog is barking, but he is barking at clouds and butterflies, not at burglars and intruders."

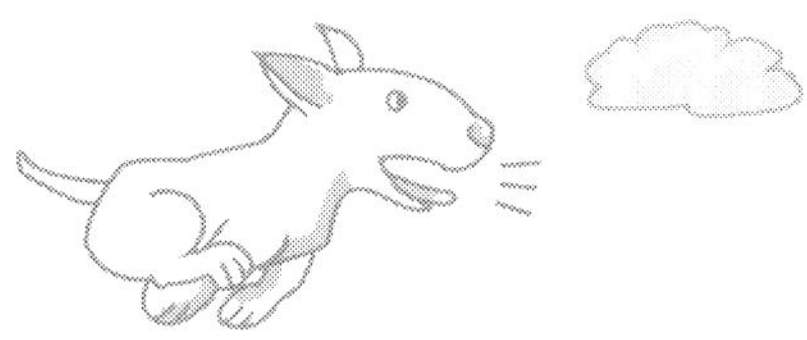

We have looked at how pain is created. We can see that:

1. Pain does not necessarily indicate that the body is damaged.
2. Pain can be learned, but this learning is *un*conscious.
3. Fear especially, can affect how much pain we feel.

This information helps us to choose treatments and resolve pain. It also increases our choice of treatments.

- We could use drugs to change brain chemistry (but they may not work and they cause additional side effects).
- We can use body therapies to change our brain patterning.
- We can learn relaxation and reassure ourselves to calm an overactive nervous system.

8

ILLUSIONS AND INTEROCEPTION

Two tactile illusions

I have included these here because I want to demonstrate how easy it is to confuse the brain.

This first one is an easy tactile illusion to try at home.

1) A hot or cold coin illusion

This experiment shows how the brain can muddle up signals of hot and cold.

You can try it on someone else, or on yourself. I find this illusion works perfectly on most people.

Take three larger coins of the same size.

Place one coin in the fridge and put the other two coins in some hot, but not boiling, water. The temperature difference does not have to be very extreme.

The coins will change temperature quickly, so you don't have to wait long.

Then place your coins in a line on a plate, with the cold one in between the two hotter ones.

Your participant (or you) places three middle fingers of one hand on the coins at the same time – one finger on each coin.

Now ask: "What temperature are the coins?"

They/you are unlikely to notice the colder middle coin; they will all feel the same temperature.

Then ask them to take their fingers off the coins and use one thumb to test each coin individually. They should now be able to tell which of the coins are hot or cold.

This illusion can help people to understand how easy it is for everyone's brain to make a mistake about sensation signals. The sensory signals from the hand to the brain are correct but the brain misinterprets the signals and tells you that the coins are all the same temperature.

2) The rubber hand

This experiment shows how our body map (schema) can be susceptible to 'drift'. This illusion works on about 80% of people.

For the rubber hand illusion, you need a rubber glove, an elastic band, a piece of cardboard, two small brushes (toothbrushes), and someone to help you.

Blow up the glove and tie it with the elastic band so it looks a bit like a hand. Then place one of your hands, and the rubber glove, palm down on a table in front of you. Cover the end of the rubber glove with a piece of clothing, so that it looks as if it is one of your hands, and use the cardboard to cover your real hand.

Then get your helper to stroke your hidden hand, and the rubber glove hand, at the *same* time in the *same* places. You can also do this with two small brushes like toothbrushes.

The participant should only be able to see the rubber glove, and if they are susceptible to the illusion it starts to look/feel like the rubber hand is their *own* hand. This is called 'body schema drift', as the brain starts to include things in its map of the body that should not be there, like a fake hand.

The opposite effect can happen in people after amputations. They can continue to experience the missing limb as if it is still attached to them. In this case, the brain is slow to update the body schema map to understand that the limb is not there now.

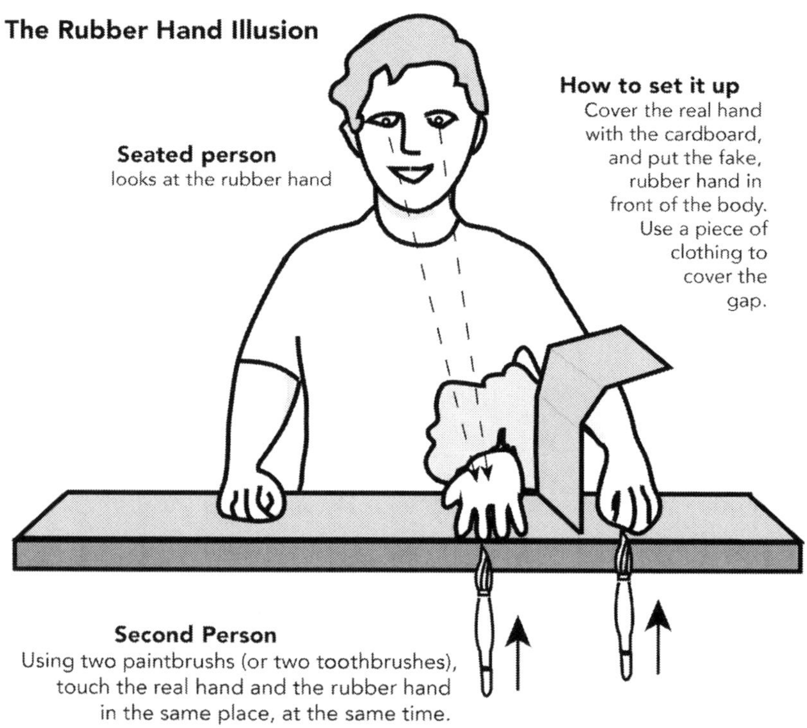

If you would like to watch a three-minute video of someone having the rubber hand illusion done to them, search for '*The Rubber Hand Illusion – Horizon: Is Seeing Believing?*' on Youtube.

Helpful illusions

You might be thinking that this 'interpretation' effect in the brain only happens when things go wrong, but actually everyone's brain is making interpretations all day.

We can literally see this blurring effect at work when we look around us because there is a blind spot in our vision.

Our eyes have a small area on the retina where we cannot reflect light, which should really give us a small dark spot in our vision. However, our brain fills in the blind spot with things it thinks *should* be there, so we never see or experience the small hole in our visual field! This is an example of our brain making *interpretations* about reality.

The following easy illusion will show you how normal it feels for your brain to give you an 'interpretation' of reality.

Perfect illusion

For this, we need two paper 'dots'.

Take some paper and tear off two very small pieces, only about the size of a quarter of your little fingernail.

Put them on a table or surface in front of you so that they are side by side and a little over a hand's width (5–6 inches) apart. It helps if the surface you use is slightly dark coloured or textured, like wood. (Don't use a clean white sheet of paper).

Now close one eye and look at the paper dot on the opposite side (if you are looking with your left eye, look at the right-hand dot). Slowly experiment with moving your face closer to the dots and keep staring at one dot.

At a certain distance, the other dot will look like it has disappeared.

You can do this with the other eye too; if you are looking with your *right* eye, look only at the *left-hand* dot and move slowly closer to the dots.

Demonstrating the 'blind spot' with paper dots

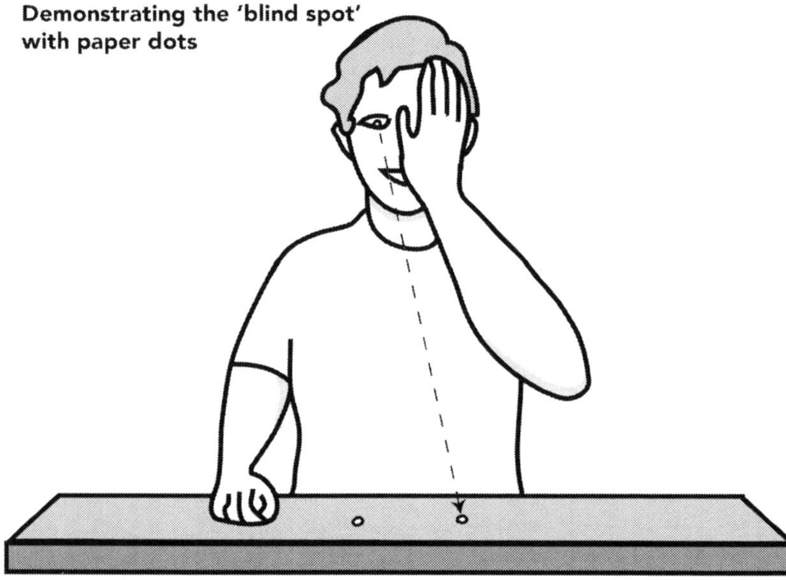

* Cover one eye
* Stare at the paper dot (the opposite one from your eye)
* Slowly lower your head towards the dots
* Keep staring at the dot, and at a certain distance the other dot will disappear but the colour of the table under the dot is 'filled in' and created by the brain.

This occurs because the blind spot on the eyes has covered the dot you are not looking at, and your brain simply isn't interested enough in a small spot to keep creating it.

If you do the same thing again, notice this time that nothing happens to the surface of your table at all, and only the paper dot disappears! This shows how fickle the brain can be with information. If the brain was telling the complete truth then the *surface of the table*, as well as the paper dot, should disappear. Instead, only the paper dot disappears!

Our brain *interprets* what is around us. This interpretation effect is the same with *all* of our sensory information including pain and other sensory interpretations. The blind spot illusion works on everyone who can see, because every sighted person's brain is interpreting visual information so that it makes 'sense'. This is what our brain does for us – it interprets reality in order to keep us safe.

Our brains have a lot of information to process, in order to create a sense of reality. To manage this, we know that our brain tends to predict that most things will stay the same and pays attention only to things that have changed or are new.

A table is a solid structure, and the brain expects it to stay put. However, the small paper dots could easily blow off the table and are not permanent, so your brain is not worried about the paper dot disappearing when your visual blind spot covers it. However, the brain can see a lot of table and it predicts (guesses) that the table does not have holes in it, so it keeps on showing you a continuous table surface with no missing areas.

Illusions as treatments

Interestingly, the rubber hand illusion has been used as a pain relief treatment for arthritis and many other types of pain, for years[1].

When this illusion is used as a movement therapy, for instance for arthritis of the hand, the illusion is set up as described above but using an *articulated* rubber hand, which has rubber fingers that can be stretched or straightened. The brain sees the movement of the rubber hand and feels no pain. Because the brain is fooled into feeling that the rubber hand might belong to the body, it reprogrammes the movement neurotags for that hand, and this causes a reduction of pain afterwards when the person moves their own hand.

This proves that even with actual physical damage, like joint damage in arthritis, the *amount* or intensity of pain is created in the brain, and we can reduce pain signals by reprogramming our body and brain coordination.

The more susceptible the person is to the rubber hand illusion, the better this kind of illusion will also work as a pain treatment. This is good news for fibromyalgia sufferers because people with fibromyalgia have been proved to be much more susceptible to this particular illusion than people without fibromyalgia[2]. This is why I am recommending brain-body reprogramming, using body-based therapies, for fibromyalgia.

A map of me

So how does our body schema, or body map, get created?

The brain creates a body map as it develops in childhood. Children develop the ability to recognise themselves in a mirror by about age four, but studies show that from four up to about the age of ten, children are more likely to use sight as a reference, rather than internal cues like proprioception (knowing where the body is located without looking at it).

So, it seems that our body schema may not be fully developed until we are around eleven years old[3].

We know that a feeling of body ownership and personal agency is critical to developing a clear body schema. A clear body map allows us to be in touch with our internal body feelings, like thirst and hunger, and it also includes our emotional feelings.

The amount of time needed to develop a complete and clear body map becomes significant when we look at how body mapping could be disrupted in childhood.

Fibromyalgia sufferers are more susceptible to the rubber hand illusion than people without fibromyalgia, which may indicate that in fibromyalgia the body maps are not as clear as they could be. We can briefly explore why this might be true.

As a child grows up feeling safe, and living free from fear, this child learns to enjoy their internal cues and to listen to them. This interior sense is called interoception.

Interoception

Interoception has been described as our eighth sense. We have five *external* senses; touch, sight, hearing, taste and smell. And three *internal* senses; proprioception (body awareness), interoception (internal body signals), and balance. Interoceptive feelings, like knowing where your feet are without looking at them, would include knowing if we are hungry or thirsty, if we are hot or cold, if our heart is beating fast, if we need to urinate, or if we are sleepy.

Fear shuts down the brain's internal cues, especially information from our digestion. For instance, we know that the digestion sends information along our vagus nerve, but this only happens well in the *Rest and Digest* state.

When we are fearful or stressed, we remain alert to the *outside* world in order to stay safe, and we suppress inside information from the gut.

You can practice using your interoception sense by watching and noticing your breathing.

Feeling and counting your own heartbeat (without taking your pulse with your hands) is another a good way to practice interoceptive awareness.

Blurry maps

It is possible that disruptions to the development of the body map can happen in childhood due to violence, fear, or abuse or even just stress. Fear alters the way the brain takes in information. A child growing up in fear would need to pay more attention to his or her outside world[4], and feelings of internal anxiety would be suppressed.

Evidence shows this to be true. People who have had lived through 'adverse childhood experiences' (ACEs) show changes to their body maps[5].

Studies done specifically with people with chronic pain show that they are statistically more likely to have had an early life adversity *and* have blurry body mapping[6].

So, we can easily demonstrate and experience body-map-blurring using our two tactile illusions. These illusions demonstrate how easily the brain is fooled, how feedback loops can be created, and how the *imprecision hypothesis of pain* works in real life.

We can also see that other kinds of body pain, ones with a visible known cause, like arthritis, have some element of incorrect body mapping. This is significant for us as it demonstrates that blurry-body-mapping, causing chronic pain neurotags, can easily occur with *other* kinds of painful illness and that it is not only a feature of fibromyalgia.

I very much hope that taking this quick tour of neuroscience will help to clear up any daft ideas about people 'creating' pain and reassure you about what 'learned pain' really is. We have a lot of scientific evidence that details exactly how chronic pain can be created, and ideas to help us resolve it. We just need to apply it to your fibromyalgia.

Sofa training

You can start to solve those blurry maps right now.

This is a really useful brain training exercise, and it doesn't even require you to move off your sofa!

While relaxing somewhere, you can do visualisations, active daydreams, ones where you concentrate and imagine moving freely without pain. You can do active daydreaming and imagine going for walks, running, sports or dancing, all pain-free.

Imagining activities stimulates the movement pathways in your brain. Sports professionals have been using these techniques to code the correct movements in the brain for years. It's not possible to train for sporting success all day, every day, as the muscles get tired, and so athletes train their mind while relaxing on the sofa[7]. This is a form of *neurological reprogramming* (in case anyone asks!).

Active daydreaming helps reprogramme your brain.

Put as much detail as possible into these daydreams. You need to especially include lots of physical sensory details; things like how your feet feel, what surface you are walking over, what clothes are you wearing, what the weather is like, how warm or cold it is, and what the light is like.

So, let's run through a typical sofa training session.

- Get comfortable, as much as you possibly can, and choose a time of day when things are better for you.
- Think of an activity. It might be swimming, or dancing, or walking, whatever would be nice to think about. It might

just be a simple movement, like stretching your arms up to the sky.

- The next part is to imagine yourself doing this activity and not feeling any pain.
- Some people tend to imagine *watching* themselves do something rather than imagine actually doing it, so make sure you are imagining *doing* the activity, (from inside the body) not just watching yourself do it (from the outside of the body).

If you are finding it hard to imagine being pain-free, then here are a couple of ideas to try.

1. Find someone to watch on YouTube or TV who is roughly the same size or shape as you are. Now watch them doing an activity – and I mean *really* watch them carefully. Then go and lie down, relax, close your eyes and imagine being them. Imagine doing the thing they were doing.

To make it as real as possible, you can imagine wearing what they were wearing, speaking like them, or being in the place they were in and looking around at that environment.

Your brain may try to tell you that the imaginary activity is going to hurt or that it does actually hurt while you are imagining doing it. If this happens, simply reassure your brain that it can't possibly hurt, firstly because you are only imagining doing the activity, and secondly because in this exercise we have borrowed someone else's body, and this body doesn't have any pain.

2. If you prefer to imagine this as a sci-fi you can imagine that you have been given a brand-new body. This body is perfect

> and will move beautifully and smoothly in any direction you ask it to go. Try it out. Walk about, notice how your new legs and arms feel. Jump, stretch, and roll – everything in this body is strong and works smoothly when you ask it to.

Spend five to ten minutes every day doing these sofa training exercises. They will help to reprogramme your brain to create new, pain-free movement pathways.

When you finish each routine you can ask yourself: what percentage of my pain is less? You might find that there is a small improvement each time. It might take a little while but cumulatively, little by little, we can achieve a lot.

It's a bit like painting over something dark on a wall with some semi-transparent white paint. To begin with, you can still see what was underneath, but if you keep painting over the dark place in layers, eventually it will be all white.

Even if you are in a lot of pain right at this moment, in the future, when you look back at that pain, you can know that you made a positive decision to find a new direction, to move to a new place in your life, and feel healthy.

Graded Motor Imagery (GMI)

This is another new technology designed to help the brain recode movement pathways, so that they become clearer and pain free. It has been developed by two leading pain scientists, Lorimer Moseley and David Butler, as part of their *Explain Pain* programme.

GMI has three parts. Firstly, it trains the brain to recognise left and right. This helps to clarify those blurry body maps for us.

There are smartphone apps that turn this into a bit of a game. For instance, a GMI exercise might show you a picture of a hand and then ask you to recognise whether it is a picture of a *right* hand or *left* hand. To answer this question, your brain has to access your own body maps to compare the picture to, and so this is a good exercise to develop clearer body maps.

Secondly, it uses imagined movement – which we have just done in our sofa training routines.

The third tool in GMI, uses mirror box therapy, which is very similar to the rubber hand illusion. Mirror box therapy works best on injuries on individual limbs, (because mirror box therapy requires you to have one limb that doesn't hurt). For this reason, it isn't so useful for widespread pain, and I won't go into the details of it here.

Interestingly, though, chronic pain can alter the way our brain processes movement, and actually makes us slower. When the left-right recognition tests were done with people with a painful right arm, studies showed that the speed they could recognise photographs of right arms was slower[8].

The reduction in pain intensity from using GMI is maintained at follow up appointments and shows that this kind of intervention makes good changes that last.

The left-right apps are called *Recognise* in the App Store if you'd like to try them.

ROUTES OUT OF FIBROMYALGIA

9

RECAP

To recap what we have found out about fibromyalgia so far:

- We have seen that when people are exposed to acute stress or trauma the vagus nerve can activate a *Shut-Down* state, or the body remains in a hyperalert (*Alert!, Fright, Fight* or *Flight*) state. Lack of good vagal tone can directly lead to higher glutamate levels.
- If the body does not return to *Rest and Digest* in order to maintain good gut function and to repair itself, higher levels of inflammatory chemicals can be produced in the body, contributing to developing hyperalgesia and chronic pain.
- Fibromyalgia often appears to begin with actual damage to the body, an injury or surgery, and it seems the brain does not realise that the original damage is now healed. Memories from past injuries can be stored in the brain and can cause incorrect interpretations of normal, neutral (safe) sensations.
- Too many warning signals, like stress and emotions, can cause an overwhelming amount of sensory information. This

can contribute to a nervous system that does not have much resilience[1]. This can lead to body signals becoming muddled.
- We've also seen that the brain interprets signals. Pain does not necessarily mean anything is wrong with the body. The brain produces pain signals to keep us away from something or stop us from moving parts of our body. Pain is like a guard dog.

So, what can we do about all of this in order to rebalance ourselves?

Are we chasing something?

In my clinic I remind clients that biologically we are no different to our cavemen ancestors; our bodies are designed to hunt for food and sometimes to run away from animals that could eat us!

When we run fast for short distances and then sit down for a rest, our body understands that we were probably chasing, or finding, something to eat. We might have climbed a tree, which is hard work, and then we sit down to eat the thing we picked or walk home calmly with the food that we have found, to share it.

Alternatively, if we run or move all day without stopping, not eating, or maybe just grabbing something to eat on our route, our body understands that we must be in danger. We must be running away from something that might eat *us*, or our environment is now *so* dangerous that we must keep moving to get to safety! Why else would we keep going all day, when we are tired, and not stop to eat and rest?

If we are running about being busy all day and then we experience additional fear and anxiety, from emotional stresses or physical trauma, the body may interpret those extra fearful feelings as indications that we are about to be caught or that we are going to die.

You will see that there are parallels here with our modern life. But the problem is that we cannot explain to our autonomic nervous system that as modern people we may have to work long days to survive, but that we are ok, or that everyone lives like this now. Your body might simply feel threatened and unsafe.

To tell your body that you are safe, you have to show it. Taking breaks throughout the day when you can sit calmly, and eating well and slowly, are very important cues to tell your autonomic nervous system that you are not being chased or in a life-threatening situation. Eating with friends or in a comfortable environment is also a healthy activity because we are social animals, designed to live in groups for safety.

Thinking calmly or taking even short breaks from worrying thoughts by using meditation or breathing exercises also gives our bodies and minds a rest, and mini-breaks like this can allow our stress levels to naturally reduce.

Why aren't some people naturally returning to a calm state?

I believe we should see fibromyalgia as a state, rather than a disease. The autonomic nervous system has activated an emergency state because, together with the brain, the autonomic nervous system believes the body is being threatened.

Pain has been created to motivate us to *do* something[2], so what should we do?

An allergy to stress

Let's look at your autonomic system differently for a moment.

No-one says to someone who suffers with hay fever that they are 'making it up' or that they are creating psychosomatic symptoms. That's because we have a medical model which understands that there is a faulty response from their immune system to pollen. The immune system belonging to a hay fever sufferer acts as if pollen is *really* dangerous and it goes into overdrive, attempting to remove all pollen from the body. If you don't have hay fever, then your immune system remembers that pollen is harmless.

Fibromyalgia appears to be a similar pattern of incorrect danger responses. This time, the autonomic nervous system acts as if the environment is really dangerous.

For people *without* fibromyalgia, their autonomic nervous system finds some places safe and allows them to relax fully, but for people with fibromyalgia, it seems that their autonomic nervous system is always on *Alert* or in a partial *Shut-Down*.

The autonomic nervous system is acting as if it is somehow *allergic* to its environment.

Inflammation is a distress signal, sent to the brain to say that that something is wrong inside the body environment, and stress causes similar signals of distress to be sent to the brain.

We know that stress can cause our nervous system to become unregulated and to become 'unresponsive to the normal range of inputs'[3] so that our nervous system can become 'locked' in a certain pattern. It is as if the autonomic nervous system in fibromyalgia is overwhelmed and stays in a threatened response state.

However, the responses to threats are not the problem. For instance, people with post-traumatic stress disorder (PTSD) and anxiety don't actually have *heightened* responses to threats; they respond in the same range as healthy people do.

The problem is that their bodies are producing threat responses to things that are harmless or neutral.

So, we have discovered that to get back to health we need to calm the brain, reduce inflammation, and teach our autonomic nervous system that we are safe.

Food is an enormously important and useful tool for us to use, as the gut gives the brain many signals about how the body is doing via the vagus nerve. A happy and calm gut tells the brain things are ok.

Throughout the book I have mentioned that reducing inflammation is important.

In the first section, we saw how brain chemistry in fibromyalgia is disturbed, which is a kind of brain inflammation. In the second section we saw how this brain inflammation can create pain. And in the next chapter we will look at inflammation in the body.

The vagus nerve will send warning signals to the brain if there is any inflammation in our internal organs, so we will take a look at what inflammation is, and what inflammation in the body does to us.

10

INFLAMMATION AND FIBROMYALGIA

You may have been wondering, as we are now already a fair way through this book, and we have been looking at pain, when we will be getting to all the *other* symptoms of fibromyalgia. To do this, we are going to look at the effects of inflammation.

Inflammation and fibromyalgia are strongly linked. The fibromyalgia condition is characterised by brain inflammation (higher than normal glutamate levels), and additionally many of the symptoms of inflammation match up with those experienced in fibromyalgia.

In fact, almost all of the common symptoms of fibromyalgia look extremely similar to inflammation.

As you read this you might wonder why the medical profession has not said anything about inflammation being linked to fibromyalgia?

Why isn't inflammation better understood?

Inflammation can occur in one place (if someone sprains their ankle there may be heat and swelling) but it can also occur throughout the body, and if it becomes chromic it has a systemic effect, which means the *whole* body responds to it. Systemic inflammation tends to create symptoms that are diverse and widespread, as with fibromyalgia.

Medical training supports the education of specialists. Which is brilliant if you have a condition that confines itself to one system or organ, but not so good if your symptoms cover many organs and body areas.

Single-system specialists in the medical profession cannot adequately treat chronic conditions that involve multiple systems. Specialists in heart disease may know little about digestion or neurochemistry. Additionally, organs are being divided up into even smaller areas. I spoke to a client recently who had to go to two different hospitals to see two different consultants, because each one only specialised in one side of his heart. There are urgent calls for this to change, precisely because inflammation is being overlooked as a cause of multiple diseases[1].

Inflammation is now implicated as a cause (rather than the result) in conditions like cardio-vascular (heart) disease, depression, fibromyalgia, diabetes, osteoarthritis and cancer, but this connection is only just becoming apparent and our current specialist medical system is not ideally placed to understand it.

For instance, patients treated conventionally are rarely asked for a complete timeline of their physical and mental health, or asked if there was anything unusual or difficult happening in their life at the time an illness started, and yet this knowledge is invaluable to track the beginning of any disease. We can see why when we look at what happens to us when inflammation occurs.

What is inflammation?

Inflammation is something that happens when there is damage to the body's 'tissues' (things like our skin, bone, muscles, and nerves).

When there is damage, 'pro-inflammatory chemicals' are released from the tissues (like cytokines), causing heat and redness.

Some of these chemicals also cause changes to the blood capillaries causing plasma fluid to build up in the tissues. This process of fluid accumulation is the swelling we experience, and it helps our immune cells to get to the injury site.

Cytokines sound bad but they are really just messengers and some of them can attract immune cells to the area of damage, which is helpful. They are a warning, telling the brain that there is damage somewhere.

We can measure cytokines in our blood, which tells us that there is inflammation happening somewhere. Some common inflammatory cytokines found in the blood have exciting names like *IL- 1, IL-6, IL-12, IL-18, TNF-a, CRP,* and *IFN-y.*

What does inflammation feel like?

We are able to study temporary effects of inflammation by looking at vaccination effects. Vaccinations trigger an inflammatory effect from the immune system as our immune cells figure out what the injected pathogen is and try to kill it.

[Vaccinations are mostly made of inactive (dead or very weak) pathogens, but our immune system doesn't know that, so it gets to practise with a 'safe' version of the illness – we know that the inflammatory effects of vaccinations are coming mainly from our own immune system, not from the disease that we are being immunised from.]

Inflammation causes us to feel:

- Feverish
- Nauseous

- Lack of appetite
- Tired
- Unable to sleep well (fragmented sleep)
- Irritability
- Low mood
- Depression
- Poor concentration
- Forgetful
- Socially withdrawn

Inflammation and glutamate

Inflammation is an important cause of glutamate dysregulation in the brain, and glutamate itself causes damage and inflammation to the brain cells[2].

I said earlier that increases in glutamate can cause chemical feedback loops to occur in the brain. When there is inflammation, the astrocyte cells in our brain (the glutamate recycling ones) react to the cytokines (inflammation messengers). This stops the astrocytes from being able to transport or recycle their normal amount of glutamate, and so glutamate levels start to increase. This increase in glutamate over-activates the glutamate receptors (the NMDA receptors), causing a circuit dysfunction in the brain cells[3].

In other words, if we have central heating or air conditioning in our house, and the thermostat goes wrong, the temperature in the building could get more and more uncomfortable. This is what happens in our brain when glutamate recycling doesn't happen properly.

I'm going to list a few common symptoms of fibromyalgia and how inflammation relates to them, and then we can look at what we can do about it.

Depression

We know inflammation can cause depression[4]. Some medical treatments for cancers use injections of pro-inflammatory cytokines (like IFN-a), which are known to cause up to 50% of patients to suffer a major depressive episode as a result. It is also very common to see depression in cases of inflammatory diseases, like rheumatoid arthritis, osteoarthritis, and inflammatory bowel diseases.

Increased glutamate levels are regarded to be a cause of depressive feelings[5].

Not everyone with depression shows high glutamate levels but when serious depression is accompanied by inflammation, glutamate is seen to be significantly elevated in the brain[6].

This indicates that there is likely to be more than one way to generate depressive states in the body, but inflammation seems to be one route[7].

Brain fog

Inflammation causes a measurable slowing-down of thought, and of physical movements. Inflammation especially affects our able to focus our attention[8].

Fatigue

An increase in one common inflammatory chemical in particular (IL-6) is associated with greater frailty and disability, and creates slow walking speed, poor muscle strength, poor lower leg function, and anaemia from lack of iron[9].

TNF-a levels are seen to be high in patients with chronic fatigue syndrome.

Sleep disturbance

Cytokines can regulate sleep, which explains how our sleep cycle can get knocked out of rhythm by inflammation. The effects of inflammation are so important to the quality of our sleep that sleep apnoea and chronic restricted sleep are now considered to be inflammatory disorders.

If people are given injections of cytokines (TNF-a and IL-1) this can create symptoms associated with sleep deprivation[10], such as:

- memory problems;
- increased pain sensitivity;
- cognitive impairment;
- sleepiness;
- depression;
- fatigue;
- type II diabetes.

Early life stress

Interestingly, stress in our early life has been linked to the development of sustained inflammation in human studies[11]. This may be one route by which adverse childhood experiences (ACEs) can negatively impact our health later in life. Our bodies become primed to produce a greater inflammatory reaction or produce stress responses more quickly to later adverse events.

Listing all of this information is ok, but the point is not to find out what has *already* gone wrong but to stop it from ever getting to that point. The evidence says that if we reduce our inflammation levels, we can reduce the chances of getting these diseases.

Our natural anti-inflammatories

You'll be pleased to hear that the body has a way of controlling inflammation, and to do this it uses cortisol. Cortisol is released when our inflammation levels rise (when there are more cytokines circulating), and the cortisol tells the cells to remain calm ('don't produce any more inflammation').

Cortisol is part of our endocrine system. The endocrine system includes glands that produce hormones, like cortisol. (Other well-known hormones are thyroid hormone, which is released from the thyroid gland, or oestrogen from the ovaries.)

In our body-organisation, I like to think of the endocrine system as the mail people. The gland writes an instruction message and the hormone (the instruction message) is sent to whoever needs to hear it. All the cells in our bodies have receptors on the outside of them. Receptors are a bit like mailboxes and cells can change what mail they want to receive by changing the receptors. Cells can *increase* receptor sites (mailboxes) to increase incoming messages, or *decrease* them to reduce the incoming mail.

Cortisol has more than one job in the body and, alongside its role in reducing inflammation, our body also uses it to help us deal with stress.

Cortisol acts as a messenger for the sympathetic nervous system (the *Alert!, Flight & Fight* team), along with adrenaline. Adrenaline gets the heart working faster, and cortisol tells the body to release more sugar into the bloodstream so it can go to our muscles. Cortisol is the chemical that slows our digestion down. Cortisol gets your body system ready to run away or have a fight.

Cortisol can manage these multiple jobs fine ...until (you guessed it) the stress continues, and the body doesn't get a break.

If stress becomes continuous, we release high levels of cortisol all of the time, but then our cells get bored of hearing the same message all the time and they simply adjust to a higher level of cortisol by *reducing* the amount of receptors (mailboxes). Suddenly, we have a system that isn't allowing so much cortisol into the cells (the cells have stopped listening) and inflammation can increase.

This is the reason why we are told that reducing stress can reduce inflammation.

(Cortisol can be tested in saliva to see how high our levels are.)

Our bodies are brilliantly arranged and many of our body chemicals are used for more than one function. This is one of the reasons that adjusting our body chemistry with drugs can be effective in the short term, and why they can cause us problems (side effects) when we try and use them long term.

How to reduce inflammation

We have two ways we can deal with inflammation ourselves, firstly by doing things that can reduce it, and secondly by avoiding things that increase inflammation.

We have evidence that natural health treatments and exercises, sometimes called mind-body therapies, treatments like acupuncture, yoga and meditation, can change our body chemistry, and the cells of our body, reducing the effects of chronic stress[12]. This can be measured using gene-expression, which is a technique that shows which genes are turned on or off in our cells.

Certain acupuncture points have been shown to specifically reduce inflammation in the body. I have included these in the self help tools for you to use.

Research: a recent review looked at 2268 people using acupuncture for depression (in 29 different studies) and found acupuncture showed 'clinically relevant benefits'[13].

This review also showed that using *electro*-acupuncture did not work for depression. Electro-acupuncture is a variation on traditional acupuncture, where electrical connections are attached to the acupuncture needles. I include this information to show you that electricity is not required to make positive changes to the brain.

Taking anti-inflammatory medications for fibromyalgia

It would sound from all this, that taking anti-inflammatory medications for fibromyalgia would be useful; however, these drugs do not work to improve fibromyalgia symptoms[14].

This is not unique to fibromyalgia, as depression caused by inflammation also doesn't respond to anti-inflammatories especially well either. This may be to do with the drugs themselves; anti-inflammatory drugs are synthetic versions of cortisol, the nearest thing we can make.

Both corticosteroids and non-steroidal anti-inflammatory drugs (NSAIDs) interfere with other steroids in the body and we see unintended effects from using synthetic versions of natural body chemicals. For instance, aldosterone controls blood pressure and sodium levels in the blood, and when we use synthetic anti-inflammatories like corticosteroids they interfere with our aldosterone. This affects our kidneys, our blood pressure goes up, and fluids accumulate in the body, often giving us a characteristic puffy face. This demonstrates how different these drugs are from our natural ones, and that we should not rely on a 'diagnosis by prescription' as a foolproof method. Just because fibromyalgia does not respond to synthetic anti-inflammatory drugs does not in itself prove there is no inflammation present.

Blood tests from fibromyalgia sufferers don't usually show higher levels of inflammation markers (cytokine levels) either. However, newer research into inflammation indicates that using a wider assessment of potential cytokines could give us better options for identifying fibromyalgia. Studies are showing that people with fibromyalgia have increased levels of fractalkine and IL-8 in their cerebral-spinal-fluid (CSF)[15].

Fractalkine helps the (microglia) cells in the brain survive when their surroundings are toxic, so high levels of fractalkine may indicate to us that the brain chemistry is not within normal ranges. This cytokine is not often measured, as it requires the fluid around the brain and spinal cord to be tested, rather than just the blood.

Again, we find evidence for brain inflammation and fibromyalgia, and more scientific evidence towards a physical explanation for fibromyalgia. But, once again, it's an explanation that has been missed up to now because it is not easy to test.

11

CALMING INFLAMMATION

When we look at ways to *avoid* inflammation, one of the most important places to begin is with our food and our digestive health. We need to look at ways to reduce as much inflammation as possible from the gut.

I'm going to recommend that you avoid sugar, cheap cooking oils, and gluten to reduce your inflammation levels. Many people with fibromyalgia find benefit from avoiding these foods and I understand that it might sound extreme, but I will explain why this might be useful for you.

We are all farmers

Imagine someone came to visit you. That person, inside their clothes, is only 50% human. Only 50% of their cells are actually human cells with human DNA. The rest, the other 50% of their cells, are made up of bacteria and small life forms that live with us and inside us.

This sounds almost unbelievable but it's true! Because the human cells are much bigger and take up more space, we only see the human ones.

The little life forms who live with us are called the *microbiota*, which just means 'little life'. Our microbiota (gut bacteria) can change very quickly, in a matter of a day, because they eat what we eat. If we help our good gut bacteria, they can help us too.

I like to think of my microbiota as my gut tenants. There are many hundreds of species of them. Unfortunately, there are also other organisms in our gut that are not so friendly.

Gut pests

Yeast is generally an unhelpful life form in our gut, and it is present in all of our guts. There are many kinds of yeast, but one particular problem family are the *Candida* family. When I think of *Candida,* I always think of a bad family gang, or terrorists but, however you visualise them, this group is not friendly!

Normally the *Candida* family are kept in check by the friendly gut bacteria called *Lactobacillus*. The *Lactobacillus* and *Candida* family compete for the same space on the lining of the gut (it's a bit like turf wars).

When we eat sugars we change the balance of power in our gut, because sugars are what members of the *Candida* family eat, allowing this yeast to multiply and get out of control. One family member, called *Candida albicans,* has the annoying ability to damage our gut walls, allowing food molecules to escape into our blood stream, which can create inflammation and allergies, and it causes problems in our organs too.

Terrorist action

We often encounter *Candida albicans* in our lives because it is the most common cause of fungal urinary tract infections (UTIs) and it is the problem that creates genital 'thrush' (also called a yeast infection).

However, the *Candida* family isn't just uncomfortable, some of them can be dangerous agents of systemic infections in immunocompromised people, like the elderly or cancer patients.

Candida can travel around the body using our bloodstream as a transport system. It can reach our brain, our eyes, our heart, in fact any internal organ can be affected. Once it has escaped the confines of the gut and is at large in the body, our next line of defence is the immune system. Our immune system has to take on the job of doing battle with the *Candida*, to keep it under control. In some cases, we can use anti-fungal drugs to knock it back but if there are still places in our gut where it can escape, it can just get out again.

Some of the less common members of the *Candida* family (*Candida auris*) have developed immunity to anti-fungal drugs and are creating havoc in hospitals all over the world.

The great escape

The common *Candida albicans* (which we all carry in our gut) lives in two forms. Mostly it lives in our gut, minding its own business and not causing problems. Our gut is pretty well defended; it's got a good layer of friendly bacteria, then there is a layer of protective mucus, and then there is the gut wall itself.

However, if the *Candida* gets hold of enough ammunition (sugars) it can multiply, and it can change shape and grow roots. I'm not using a metaphor here; it really does grow actual roots called *hyphae*, and it uses these roots to get through our gut wall.

Candida is unusual because it is even able to change the surrounding Ph levels (acid or alkaline) to a level that it likes, so that it can then change into the root growing stage[1].

I'm sure you are not enjoying the sound of all this, and neither do our bodies.

Collateral damage

Candida albicans has the ability to increase any inflammation that it finds. If there is some inflammation from a small amount of damage in the gut, let's say you ate something that didn't agree with you, then *Candida albicans* can take advantage of the chaos and colonises that area. Once it is living there, it is capable of delaying healing and so it exacerbates the original problem. This allows it to either take over more space or to escape through the gut wall into the bloodstream and gain access to the rest of our body.

For instance, we know that when it is in the stomach, *Candida albicans* colonises gastric ulcers and makes them more likely to perforate (bleed). It can also increase our blood levels of the cytokines IL-17 and IL-23 and is frequently found in people with inflammatory bowel diseases[2].

More underhand tactics

Candida is a really old enemy for humanity and our bodies have been doing battle with it for centuries. Over that time, those little terrorists have developed a sneaky trick to get us to eat sugar, to keep them alive and fuel their destructive habits.

If we don't eat much sugar, or many refined carbohydrates that will digest into sugar very quickly, then the *Candida* will simply die. They can't live on anything else. When they die, they produce chemicals that are uncomfortable for us, things like tiny amounts of ethanol and other chemicals. We might experience mild symptoms like headaches or tiredness from the *Candida* dying off, but what we are most likely to experience are sugar cravings.

Our clever immune system has worked out that the foods that stop these symptoms are carbohydrates and sugars, but unfortunately our immune system doesn't realise that these foods are for the *Candida* to eat again!

So, the *Candida* has tricked our body into creating a sugar craving to keep itself alive and well fed! If you have sugar cravings then bad yeasts are holding you to ransom, 'either you eat some sugar, or we will all die and make you feel unwell'!

Fortunately, it doesn't take long for *Candida* to die off; in a few days the amount can reduce drastically. The gut will take longer than that to re-populate, so we need to maintain a sugar-free diet for several months while the gut heals and develops good populations of friendly bacteria.

Fortunately, once we reduce our sugar intake, the *Candida* will go back to safe levels, and our sugar cravings reduce too. Sweet things are nice, but they should be small treats, not a kind of food we eat regularly or to excess.

Candida is extremely common. It is likely that we all have a bit of candida that has escaped our gut and is hanging out somewhere. If our blood sugar is high, then the Candida is waiting in our blood stream to take advantage of this. We know that people with diabetes are at greater risk of getting conditions like thrush if they do not manage their blood sugars very well and the sugar in their blood increases. A sugar rush is like a big party for your resident *Candida.*

Things that encourage Candida overgrowth:

- Sugar – like sweets, ice cream, chocolate, and excessive fruit in the diet.
- Oestrogens and synthetic Oestrogens – including the contraceptive pill, HRT, and pregnancy.
- Steroids – because steroids depress our immune system, which is fighting the *Candida* for us.
- Alcohol – which causes inflammation in our organs, and alcohol digests into sugar.
- Antibiotics – which kill off our useful *Lactobacillus,* leaving our gut lining ready for invasion.**
- Diets that are too high in refined carbohydrates – like white flour products, cake, biscuits, pasta, and bread. This kind of diet needs to be changed to include more proteins, vegetables, and good oils and fats.

** Antibiotics are designed to kill bacteria and they also kill off our gut bacteria. This leaves our gut without its protective *Lactobacillus* helpers and *Candida* takes over more space on the lining of the gut. This is why using antibiotics can leave us vulnerable to thrush and UTIs, and why you should take probiotics to try to re-populate your gut after taking antibiotics.

Vitamin supplements that are recommended to help get rid of *Candida* are N-Acetyl Cystine (NAC) which sounds very chemical but is just an amino acid, and Caprylic Acid which is made from coconuts.

Gut health and fibromyalgia

The brain is very interested in how our gut feels. Our gut sends signals to the brain via the vagus nerve. Eating sugars increases the amount of *Candida* in our body, which increases inflammation.

Candida does not directly cause fibromyalgia. *Candida* does, however, cause inflammation to increase, and it especially causes gut inflammation. Most of this inflammation is probably 'sub-clinical', meaning that it isn't enough on its own to cause a disease, but we can clearly see that *Candida* is another unhelpful burden on the body and especially on our immune system.

If fibromyalgia was caused by one thing then we would have worked out what we need to avoid and probably solved the condition a long time ago. Unfortunately, however, fibromyalgia is an accumulation of stresses; things gradually becoming out of balance in the body over time until there is a tipping point and we start to see specific symptoms of glutamate increases, and widespread symptoms all over the body.

Biomedical scientists in Italy have researched the affect of diet and recommend a low sugar, low fructose diet for fibromyalgia[3].

We already have a good natural system to keep this pest under control, with good diet and our good gut bacteria. Look after them, and don't feed *Candida.*

The sugar we are eating

Sugar that is naturally part of the food you eat, like the sugar in an apple or a carrot is not a problem, because the fibre in fruit and vegetables helps the gut digest the sugars slowly.

However, if we make apple juice from that apple the sugars are more free to cause problems. If the apple juice is processed even more, into pure fructose (fruit sugar), then it can become unhealthy for us to consume. The more something sweet is processed, the quicker the sugar can be released from the food into our blood.

Even a small amount of these pure (freed) sugars cause inflammation in the body. In a study in Switzerland, 29 men aged between 19–25 added one can of sugar sweetened drink (like a can of fizzy drink) to their diet. Fizzy drinks are often sweetened with fructose. After only three weeks the men developed increased inflammation markers in their blood[4]. It is not normal for inflammation levels in the blood to suddenly rise, so this was a very worrying result.

Sweetened fizzy drinks are no good for anyone, not even in small amounts.

Fruit juice isn't great either (whatever the carton says) and should be drunk very sparingly or not at all. We can't tell how much fruit we have eaten when it is juiced, and we tend to overdo it. Not many of us would want to sit down and eat three apples, a banana, half a mango, and a pear in one sitting, but many of could enjoy drinking that lot as a smoothie. Eating whole fruit is much better for us, as long as we don't over do it.

Remember that *Candida* doesn't care what kind of sugar you provide it with, it likes them all.

Water everywhere

Water is a good anti-inflammatory, but I have heard some people say that they don't like drinking water.

If someone invited you to join a religious cult, a cult that would take money from you and make you sick, you'd sensibly say, "No way!" But if you regularly drink fizzy drinks or anything other than natural plain water, then you've already joined. Your taste buds have been brainwashed, indoctrinating you into believing that fluids should be flavoured, and then you keep giving money to someone to sell it to you.

Humans are designed to drink water.

Diet drinks

Sugar-filled drinks are obviously bad, but artificial sweeteners are no good either. They are not telling your digestion the truth; they fool it into thinking that (actual) sugar is arriving in the stomach, but then no sugar arrives.

We need to get your gut and your brain talking to each other clearly. If you allowed a child to put sweets in their mouth but not to ever swallow one, you'd soon end up with a pretty annoyed and confused child. Your body needs to be looked after, and you are in charge.

There is research to back this recommendation. In 2014, the respected journal *Nature*, published a study showing how artificial sweeteners created glucose intolerance (diabetes) by altering our gut microbiota[5].

Shortly afterwards in 2015, the *British Medical Journal* published a report that said: '*Artificially sweetened beverages and fruit juice showed positive associations with incidence of type 2 diabetes*[6]*.*'

If artificial sweeteners are part of a group of chemicals that can increase diabetes, then they are messing, at a fundamental level, with the way our brain and gut function together.

Fruit is ok, isn't it?

Yes, in moderation. Keeping to one piece a day maximum is a good plan, and if you eat a second portion try to keep mainly to lower sugar fruits, like berries.

Fructose, the sugar in fruit, can be especially a problem for people who are overweight or insulin resistant (diabetic type II) as it is digested differently to glucose.

Sugar

The conclusion is really that all sugar should only be eaten in small quantities. How small? The World Health Organisation (WHO) recommend a daily intake of no more than 30g total sugar intake per day which is about seven teaspoons of sugar. In Europe, you can look up the amounts of sugar in foods on the packets.

Most labels will give you the amount per 100g, so that the amount of sugar they say is in 100g is the same as a percentage. A tomato pasta sauce that has 6.8g of sugar in 100g is 6.8% sugar. That might not sound too bad, but it means that the whole 500g jar contains 32.4g. (6.8 x 5) which is eight teaspoons of sugar. Sugar is present in foods that sound natural too; a litre of cow's milk contains 50g of sugar (as lactose, a naturally occurring sugar in animal milk) which is over 12 teaspoons.

Sugar, along with things like modified starch, gelatine, and milk whey powders are often added to processed (packet) foods because they are cheap fillers. Instead of paying for cheap (padded out) foods that create profits for factory owners, instead aim to cook 'from scratch' when you can and try to make sure that any packet foods that you buy is low in sugar and 'non-food' ingredients.

Spare person

We need to address our excess body fat to reduce our inflammation levels. I know this isn't a popular topic, so I'll keep it short. Body weight is a rough marker, so it's a useful place to start, but it doesn't tell us everything. Body fat is the bit we need to adjust – not weight.

So, what is the problem with having a bit of extra fat?

Body fat, also called *adipose tissue,* is not all fat cells. It is actually made up of fat cells plus many immune cells. Those immune cells, called macrophages, respond to inflammation anywhere in the body and they join in with any inflammation process.

High levels of body fat are associated with low-grade, chronic inflammation because the fat itself can create cytokines, like TNF-a, IL-6 and IL-8, which is why obesity is itself classed as an 'inflammatory condition'. The good news is that if you eat a good diet and lose all the packaged meals, processed foods and sugary sweets, your weight is very likely to start to normalise for your body frame.

Oils that are good for us

We need to eat good quality oils in our diet. Excluding all fats from our diet is not healthy, and it is problematic that for years people have been told to buy low-fat processed products instead of good-quality, natural foods.

Our diets need to contain good fats and oils because our nerves and our brain are made of them. Without good fats, the body simply runs out of materials to build and repair the brain and nervous system with. If we eat poor quality fats (like frequently heated oils found in fried take-away and packaged foods) then our brain will be constructed from poor-quality materials. Frequently heated and over refined oils are a known cause of inflammation.

Choose cold pressed, extra virgin, or organic oils for cooking and making salad dressings. Avoid margarines and all refined oils. Oils that are especially bad for us are soybean oil[7], canola (rapeseed) oil, palm oil, and corn oil.

Organic butter is a natural product, whereas margarines and

'spreadable butters' are full of cheap refined vegetable oils. Instead of eating butter, you could take up the european habit of dipping bread in fresh olive oil. Extra-virgin olive oil has been shown to increase memory and improve brain health[8]. Be careful to only buy extra virgin olive oil, as much of the oil for sale in supermarkets is mixed with cheap refined olive oil which is no good. Refined oils have been heat-treated. Coconut oil is another good option for an oil to cook with.

Fish oils are good and can be taken in supplements or eaten in oily fish. Fish oils have been shown to be anti-inflammatory, especially for the brain[9]. They help to improve depression and arthritis.

Flaxseed oil is also a good source of omega-3 fats which most of us are deficient in. Flaxseed or hemp oils cannot be heated or cooked with, so eat them in cold dressings or pour over food.

A protein to be wary of

Approximately 1% of all people are suspected to be allergic to gluten, which is a protein found in some of the grains that humans eat, and most of these people will be diagnosed (often in childhood) because they developed a severe digestive problem. This condition is called 'coeliac'. If your body has an allergy to something, it creates an antibody to that substance, and people with coeliac disease have antibodies to gluten in their blood.

However, it seems that many people can be *mildly sensitive* to gluten, and they might not show severe digestive problems. Normally only people diagnosed with a severe bowel or digestive problem are tested for gluten allergy, but recent gluten testing done for people with other illnesses showed surprising results:

- 57% of people with a 'neurological illness with no known cause' had antibodies to gluten.

- 41% of people with neurodegenerative diseases had antibodies to gluten.

40% of people with peripheral neuropathy had antibodies to gluten[10].

These are very high numbers. Many doctors are now pointing to gluten as a potential health risk for neurological diseases affecting the brain[11]. Gluten antibodies are inflammatory to the brain, and the cytokines produced by this inflammation are damaging to brain tissue.

Gluten sensitivity has been shown to cause difficulties with concentration, chronic headaches, learning difficulties, bone or joint pain, muscle cramps, leg numbness, weight loss, chronic fatigue, autism, anxiety and 'brain fog'.

Studies show significant success is possible, to improve the symptoms of fibromyalgia by removing all gluten from the diet[12]. This is empirical evidence, which means it is evidence from individual people, not from a study.

Combining this information, with the new evidence we have connecting gluten with neurological illnesses, makes a strong case for removing all gluten from our diet to help with fibromyalgia.

Gluten free

Wheat, rye, spelt, and barley contain gluten. Oats do not contain gluten, but if they are rolled, they can come into contact with gluten from other grains in the factory.

Giving up gluten doesn't sound like much fun, but the gluten-free pastas are generally acceptable. Gluten free bread isn't so wonderful but going gluten-free will stop you from eating many things that are not ideal for a good diet anyway, like cake.

A gluten-free diet encourages us to eat from a wider variety of options like buckwheat, which is not actually a wheat (and makes good pancakes), quinoa, amaranth, rice (look for Italian or French rice if you don't like the Asian rice varieties), and potatoes and yams are still fine to eat. Making our own food products and meals can be more rewarding than buying factory-made ones.

Be aware when you are buying gluten-free products that Xanthan Gum can cause some people to experience IBS and gut irritation that can last a week or more. It is used as a thickener and has the code E415 in the UK and Europe. Many of the 'gum' thickeners in foods, like Xanthan Gum and Carrageenan are known gut irritants. They are put into all kinds of processed foods from sauces, cakes, puddings, many gluten-free products and even plant-based processed foods like dairy-free custard or cream may contain them, so watch out.

Overall, the evidence for a gluten-free diet has been very confusing and not definitive. A recent review of clinical studies pointed out that only one study actually looked at changes in gut microbiota from avoiding gluten. This study highlighted that the microbiota in people with a non-coeliac gluten intolerance (NCGS) seemed to be more sensitive to changes in the diet than other people who had no symptoms from eating gluten.

I believe it is worth adopting a gluten-free diet and seeing if it helps you. If giving up all gluten for six weeks does not give you a noticeable improvement in your health, then there is no health benefit from continuing to avoid gluten. If this is the case, then I recommend looking instead at the FODMAP system.

FODMAPs

FODMAPs are six groups of *short chain sugars*, but these are not the sweet kind of sugar that we were taking about earlier. These are indigestible sugars. If you are a horse, then grass tastes sweet, especially in the summer, and it can contain up to 45% sugar that a horse can taste and digest. However, to you and I, grass is not edible and does not taste sweet. FODMAP sugars are like the sugars in grass; they are indigestible by humans and, in some people, they cause all kinds of digestive problems.

FODMAPs are recognised by the medical profession. The system removes certain aggravating food groups from your diet, and it is growing as a recommendation for gut related issues. Ask your doctor to be referred to a dietician who will work out which foods may be aggravating your digestion.

What about dairy?

This is one of those areas where science can't give us a definitive answer. Yes, cows milk contains hormones like oestrogen and progesterone, lots of them, but bovine hormones are nearly all inactivated by our liver. Only about 10% of bovine progesterone is potentially active in humans, but there is evidence for bovine estradiol increasing some cancers in humans[13].

Humans may have eaten animal milks for centuries, but modern dairy cows are required to become pregnant while still lactating (producing milk) for six months of their pregnancy, increasing the oestrogen in their milk. Dairy is big business – the average value of UK dairy exports is £1.3 billion every year. Cows naturally live for 20–25 years, but being a commercial dairy cow is stressful and they are lucky to make it to seven years old before dying.

I'm not going to tell you that you must give up dairy, but I will recommend you eat a lot less of it as we really don't know the effects that eating large or regular amounts has on adults. I would highly recommend you go completely dairy free for at least two months to see if anything changes, and if anything changes when you re-introduce it.

Lactose intolerance is common but you can get tested for this if you want to be sure. If you are lactose intolerant, the undigested lactose (a type of sugar) gets into your intestines, upsets your gut bacteria and, among other things (like loose stools, gas, bloating, or mucus), it also makes your poo acidic, which can be easily tested by your doctor.

Dairy gets into all kinds of food, from bread, crisps, and crackers to sauces, puddings, and ready meals. Dried milk powder and whey are commonly used as bulking agents in processed foods.

If you are looking for substitutes, be aware that not all soya is healthy. Traditional soy foods are fermented, like tofu, tempeh, miso and the sauces tamari and shoyu. Modern soy foods are made with an isolated soy protein and it is turned into soy milk, soy cheese, soy yoghurt, and ice cream. This kind of soy protein also gets put in bread and meat products to bulk them out. It can contain chemicals such as hexane, which is used to produce it, and has been shown to lower thyroid function in some people. For these reasons, I would keep non-fermented soy foods to a minimum and only buy organic soy.

Take care with all dairy substitution foods; they might look 'natural' and plant based but they are still processed and some of them may contain gums, flavourings, and modified starches which can all irritate the gut.

What will I notice from changing my diet?

As a practitioner, I would like to point out that bloating, gas, belching, rumbling or squealing noises, discomfort of any kind, mucus or blood around your poo (a poo is called a *stool* in medicine), and anything other than at least one soft but well-formed poo a day (for instance, any constipation or diarrhoea) is not healthy. We are aiming for a calm and happy gut that does not complain at all, whatever your age.

I am lactose intolerant, which means I can't eat dairy and I do understand the feeling of looking at a food that I would really like to eat, but instead making the decision to avoid it, and choosing something else in order to look after my gut and my health. Having a healthy body on the inside is a lovely feeling, and I really encourage you to do everything you can to help your digestion.

12

OTHER CAUSES OF INFLAMMATION

You could probably guess that smoking is inflammatory. Smoking has also been shown to increase pain sensitivity in fibromyalgia[1]. Vaping might have a lower cancer risk, but it causes damage to vital immune cells and creates inflammation.

I would recommend that if you still drink alcohol, you do so very sparingly.

It's also worth reducing household pollutants. Household fragrances are just chemicals you don't need to breathe. The same applies to candles, which are mostly made of paraffin, which when burnt pollutes the air in your home with several known carcinogens and soot. Human perfumes are also heavy on chemicals and are not a good product to put directly on your skin.

Common allergies

In 2013, a study was done at Stockholm University in Sweden, in which fifteen women with fibromyalgia were tested for metal allergies.

Every single one of them was found to be allergic to at least one kind of metal[2].

All the women were re-interviewed five years later and half the women in the study were cured of fibromyalgia simply by removing exposure of the metal they were allergic to. This was not a very big trial, and there are not many studies done on metal allergies, however metal allergy testing is cheap and reliable.

If you have a reaction to metal exposure, the resulting inflammation could cause an increase in glutamate levels.

- Metals occur in many places in our environment and allergies to them are common.
- Lead and manganese are known to prevent glutamate recycling and can cause increased glutamate levels[3].
- Approximately 20% of the population are allergic to nickel.
- Smoking both passively or actively can pollute your body with nickel.
- Living near a road, factory, airport, or crematorium can increase your exposure to metals.
- Alcohol and smoking negatively impact the mechanisms affecting brain chemistry[4]

Nickel is commonly found in cosmetics, along with lead. Jewellery that is not gold or silver often contains nickel (be aware that in gold or silver-*plated* jewellery, nickel is often underneath the plating). Piercings often contain nickel.

Some people are sensitive to gold or silver, so do not just assume that gold and silver are ok!

Titanium is also a problem for some people. Many cosmetics and sunscreens contain titanium, as do dental implants and some jewellery.

Mercury is found in amalgam fillings and in crowns.

To determine whether you have a sensitivity to metals, you can ask a healthcare profession to refer you for a MELISA test. The test currently costs US$30.

Hormones and fibromyalgia

Hormones are another potential area that can affect inflammation. Progesterone in particular is important for fibromyalgia, as it too can influence natural glutamate recycling in the body.

Progesterone is used in the bodies of both men and women as a hormone and also as a 'neuro-steroid', a brain chemical. It is so important to our health that it is synthesised in several places in the body, from our adrenals, brain, and nervous system to the ovaries in women. Men and women have similar levels of it, although women's levels fluctuate through their menstrual cycle, and progesterone levels drop slightly after menopause.

Progesterone is a very protective substance in the brain, helping to prevent strokes and neuro-generative diseases[5]. Progesterone helps us to feel sleepy and has an anti-stress effect. Myelin, the coating on many of our nerves, is also under the influence of progesterone[6]. Progesterone is also being trialled to help with substance abuse (in both men and women) as it seems to reduce cravings for cigarettes, alcohol, and recreational drugs[7].

How hormones help to regulate glutamate

Alongside its own protective effects, progesterone provides us with an important ally to regulate our glutamate levels called allopregnanolone. Our bodies convert progesterone into this important neuro-steroid.

Allopregnanolone is calming, it reduces feelings of anxiety, tension, stress, and depression and has analgesic and anaesthetic actions. It is also anti-inflammatory.

Importantly for fibromyalgia, allopregnanolone influences cellular mechanisms in the skin that transport glutamate. Low levels of allopregnanolone mean that *less* glutamate is transported and recycled[8]. Glutamate levels can then rise, both in the tissue plasma and inside the cells themselves.

The first study to really examine how hormones might affect fibromyalgia pain in women was only published in 2018. This study took daily blood samples from eight women with fibromyalgia to accurately test their natural hormone levels over a month. The researchers measured their testosterone, oestrogen, progesterone, and cortisol (a stress hormone), and they also measured the level of pain the women experienced every day. From the data, the researchers could see that the women's pain levels were lowest when cortisol was low and also that their pain levels were lowest when their progesterone levels were higher[9]. So, promoting higher progesterone and lowering our cortisol could reduce pain levels.

It is surprising that this subject has been so neglected. The only other hormone study done on women with fibromyalgia was published in 2006[10], but in that study the women were only tested three times during their menstrual cycle. From that minimal testing, the researchers in 2006 did not think that hormones affected fibromyalgia pain, but this disagrees with the conclusions from many animal studies, from which we have good evidence that hormones *do* affect pain.

Hormones in contraceptives

If you use hormone contraceptives, you will find they contain a synthetic version of progesterone called progestin. Unlike our natural progesterone, progestins can prevent ovulation, which is why they can be used as contraceptives.

However, synthetic progestin has other effects. Unlike natural progesterone, it cannot be completely converted to allopregnanolone in the body[11] [12]. These synthetic variations work differently in the central nervous system[13].

Some types of synthetic progestins are known to actually reduce our levels of allopregnanolone[14], which is not ideal because low levels of allopregnanolone are strongly correlated with depression[15] and pain sensitivity in humans[16].

Hormones are a complicated area and everybody is slightly different, so it is not possible to give you advice here that will suit everyone but it may be worth trying a non-hormonal contraceptive to see if it helps your body or alternatively try a contraceptive that uses the newer progestin Nesterone[17].

Hormone Replacement Therapy (HRT) drugs for menopause

The kind of progesterone found in Hormone Replacement Therapy (HRT) is usually the synthetic progestin called MPA. For the reasons described above, if you are using HRT, I would recommend that you find a bio-identical version of progesterone instead of MPA.

The natural, bio-identical versions of progesterone are called micronised progesterone. Bio-identical progesterone is made from plants, usually Mexican Yam or Soy. Only this bio-identical type of progesterone can be converted into allopregnanolone in the body.

Balancing hormones naturally

A good diet can help us to synthesise our hormones correctly from cholesterol. [Yes, that's right, the hormones in our body are made from cholesterol.] Contrary to what you might have heard, cholesterol is actually a healthy substance that protects the brain and nervous system!

Statin drugs that lower cholesterol have not been proved to be good for brain health, and in fact many studies show that high cholesterol is neuroprotective and is very good for our brains[18].

Unfortunately, when we eat sugars the sugar changes the structure of our lovely cholesterol so that it cannot work correctly. Instead, this sugar-altered cholesterol becomes sticky and potentially dangerous, able to clog up our blood vessels. Eating sugar means the liver creates more LDL ('bad' cholesterol). For this reason, a low sugar diet is not just better for our brain and our heart health but also for our hormones too.

Stress is a major hormone disruptor.

In response to stress the adrenals release extra doses of hormones, like progesterone and cortisol, to allow us to perform well, but this extra boost system can upset the body's balance if we use it regularly.

The affects of stress have been extensively studied in animals. We know from studies using rodents that social isolation can have dramatic effects on their hormone balance. Mice and rats that are isolated for six weeks show a 50% reduction in their allopregnanolone levels[19].

Human studies show that women who had post-traumatic stress disorder (PTSD) had only approximately a third of the allopregnanolone they should have[20], and soldiers returned from Iraq and Afghanistan with PSTD also showed significantly lower levels of allopregnanolone, which related to reported severity of chest pain and muscle soreness[21].

Allopregnanolone is another measurable indicator demonstrating the detrimental effects that stress could produce in our body.

Fortunately, the body is not static and it can change.

Progesterone levels increase in response to social interaction[22]. Hugs and comedies, closeness and trust can raise our oxytocin levels[23], and lowering our stress levels may improve our allopregnanolone also.

Magnesium helps us to produce progesterone. Some foods that are high in magnesium include dark leafy greens, seeds, nuts, dark chocolate, avocados, and bananas.

Women, men, and chronic pain

Women are more likely to be diagnosed with fibromyalgia, but women in general suffer more often with chronic states than men. We are slowly making progress towards finding out why this happens.

Microglia cells in our spinal cord are part of our pain management system, and they contribute to all chronic pain states. Some changes to microglia in the spinal cord are sex dependent. It appears that female rats switch from the microglial cells and use T-cells (immune cells) for pain sensitisation. This means that men and women may not create chronic pain the same way.

I would love to tell you more about this, but it has only just begun to be explored. Many pain studies previously only used male rats and differences in cellular processes between genders went unnoticed for some time[24].

Rheumatoid arthritis (RA), polymyalgia rheumatica (PMR), and fibromyalgia

These three diseases are all characterised by chronic pain. I am often asked about the differences between them and so it may be useful to take a very brief overview of their diagnostic differences.

Rheumatoid arthritis (RA) is an auto-immune disorder occurring when the body's immune system has switched to attacking the joints in the body. Blood tests and pain symptoms are used to diagnose it. RA is associated with smoking, and with heart and lung diseases.

It is possible to have RA and fibromyalgia. These RA patients are seen to have less inflammation in their joints but experience greater pain than people who only have RA.

Polymyalgia rheumatica (PMR) is not so easily diagnosed and, like fibromyalgia, polymyalgia also lacks a standard classification criteria. However, if elevated levels of inflammatory cytokines are found in blood tests these inflammation markers are used as a diagnostic tool (blood tests may show elevated IL-6, CRP & ESR).

Polymyalgia rheumatica (PMR) is more common in older than younger people, generally over 50, and mainly in those over 70 years old and is the most common inflammatory rheumatic disease in the elderly.

PMR is characterised by pain at the shoulder and hip, accompanied by fatigue, global pain, morning stiffness, and mental function impairment in a very similar pattern to fibromyalgia, although the pain in fibromyalgia is considered to be more extreme.

One of the main differences between PMR and fibromyalgia, is that PMR comes on suddenly.

The most popular empirical ('try-it-and-see') diagnostic tool used by clinicians to diagnose PMR is to look for a positive response to corticosteroid drugs (such as Prednisone)[25]. If there is a 50% improvement in symptoms from the use of corticosteroids, then polymyalgia is diagnosed. (Even if the patient initially responds well to the steroids, some people will still experience a relapse.)

Some people are diagnosed with PMR but have normal blood results and chronic pain, but then later develop elevated inflammatory markers in blood tests. One study done in the Netherlands showed that this occurs in about 50% of polymyalgia cases[26]. This poses interesting questions about the length of time someone could be symptomatic i.e. chronic pain *without* inflammatory markers, (which sounds like fibromyalgia), before developing inflammatory markers and being diagnosed with PMR. The sudden onset of symptoms is the only clinical difference between the two conditions for some clients.

We know that inflammation naturally increases as we age, especially after 50 years old. This effect is well researched and is called 'inflamm-aging'[27]. Low levels of inflammation in our body slowly increase, our gut bacteria also change as we age, and our immune system has to work harder as more of our cells need replacing. It is possible to ask if PMR is simply the same kind of disorder as fibromyalgia, but one seen in older people and maybe as a result of an infection or a trigger event.

Fibromyalgia becomes the last option on a list of diagnostic options.

If a person with widespread joint pain coupled with psychological symptoms such as depression does not have RA markers in their blood tests, or increased levels of inflammation, and is under 50 years old, then fibromyalgia is a diagnosis that might be given.

Conditions associated with polymyalgia

Giant cell arteritis (GCA)

Up to 20% of people with PMR will also develop a condition called giant cell arteritis. This is an inflammation of the arteries, normally the ones in the head. The symptoms are fever, severe headache or soreness in the sides of the head, sudden loss of vision, irritation and redness of the white of the eye, eye pain, squints, scalp pain, or jaw pain. I am including this information here as this condition can sometimes be misdiagnosed and it needs to be treated immediately to avoid further damage or blindness.

Comparing these conditions

There are many similarities between polymyalgia and fibromyalgia, although PMR has more credibility with the medical profession. What else can we learn about fibromyalgia from looking at polymyalgia?

In general, we can say that both conditions are inflammatory diseases[28]. Blood tests for PMR are done on blood taken from the body, whereas in fibromyalgia we know that inflammation is found in the cerebral-spinal-fluids (CSF). A lumbar puncture is required to remove CSF, which is far more invasive than a blood test and so they are rarely done routinely.

We have known for decades that inflammatory chemicals induce anxiety and sickness behaviours in animal studies[29]. Studies on polymyalgia in humans demonstrate that an increase in inflammation chemicals can produce more mental-emotional symptoms[30] than physical symptoms. People with PMR who experience more pain don't necessarily have higher levels of inflammation, but the inflammation levels *are* higher in the people experiencing more mental and emotional problems. In essence, by looking at PMR we see proof that widespread inflammation in the body can make us feel unhappy and anxious.

Typically, doctors rely on blood tests from blood from the body, and no testing is done on cerebral-spinal fluids (CSF) which may be one reason why we are not seeing better diagnostics for fibromyalgia. Whilst a diagnosis will not assist anyone to get better, a useful test would give fibromyalgia the same medical validity that PMR has, hopefully assisting better research and finally giving fibromyalgia sufferers the credibility they deserve.

Chronic widespread pain

Chronic widespread pain (CWP) is the same kind of pain that fibromyalgia patients experience. It tends to be given as a diagnosis alongside another condition.

A diagnosis is just a name given to a collection of symptoms, hopefully so it can be treated and understood better. However, sometimes a diagnosis can mean that medics stop looking for the causes. A diagnosis of fibromyalgia may disguise a different condition that can contribute to the pain. For instance, early inflammatory spondyloarthritis is very similar to fibromyalgia, and patients can also experience mood and sleep changes. Up to a third of people affected by spondyloarthritis also have fibromyalgia.

In lupus also, between 20% to 40% of people with lupus also have fibromyalgia, and chronic widespread pain is common in most people who have Ehlers-Danlos and hypermobility[31].

I wanted to briefly discuss these conditions, but we should not rely too heavily on a diagnosis. Some clinicians simply do not 'believe' in fibromyalgia and may refuse to give a fibromyalgia diagnosis and send their patients away with antidepressants or painkillers (without considering the risks of these drugs), but some doctors are wisely cautious of giving a fibromyalgia diagnosis because of the risk that it may hide another condition, and because there is no reliable or simple test for fibromyalgia at the moment that will confirm a diagnosis.

NEW BEGINNINGS

13

REBOOT YOUR BRAIN

In this chapter we'll move on from inflammation and now look towards body-based therapies, for ideas we could use to reverse fibromyalgia.

Glutamate and memory

We have looked at how our brains can get muddled up if there are too many signals. We saw how neurotags mean that different things can get joined up in the brain, like a pop song and a feeling.

We can unravel the unhelpful neurotags – the ones that have combined warning signals (pain) with normal movements (even a small movement like breathing). To unravel these unhelpful neurotags we need the brain to 'forget' them.

Glutamate is involved with learning, but the brain also uses glutamate to *forget* things.

This is because memories are not really 'forgotten' or 'erased' from the mind. To forget or unlearn something, mostly we construct a *new* memory and then use this new thinking instead.

It's a bit like finding a better route to work and choosing to take the new one, rather than the old route. The old route is still there, but the new one becomes our habit.

Note: There is evidence that glutamate receptor blockers, (like pregabalin – Lyrica) prevent the brain from being able to create new memories[1], so we might not find it so easy to unlearn things while on these drugs.

How to change a memory

If an event happens more than once, the memory of it gets 'consolidated' or confirmed, so that it can be remembered more easily. We tend to revisit painful or traumatic memories in our mind in an attempt to understand them. Often simply revisiting the memory of an event over and over is not helpful, as it just creates fear. [Revisiting memories in therapy should be done so the memory becomes less fearful.]

As we know, some memory is conscious and some memory is created *un*consciously.

For example, I can remember where I live now (conscious memory), but I do not know if my brain remembers what my previous house smelt like (unconscious memory).

Memories can be strengthened, but they can *also* be weakened. Memories are not fixed and they can change.

To reduce the potency of a memory we can interrupt the 'consolidation' stage of a memory. This works even when it is a really powerful memory that we have thought about a lot or if it is a memory of something we experienced many times.

To do this firstly we need to reactivate a cue. A cue is usually a thing, a thought, an event, a memory, or just an item; anything that might trigger the memory. Then secondly, we do something differently and introduce something new into that memory.

We can do this ourselves with our thoughts by changing things like the soundtracks or the colour schemes of our memories. We often remember a static image of a memory or a short piece of time, like a piece of video. If the memory is in colour, we could make it black and white. If it is a big image, we can make it smaller and dimmer, whichever feels like it makes the memory safer or more 'friendly'. You can imagine shrinking the image, so it is tiny, like a grain of sand.

Some people prefer to change the soundtrack. We can overwrite any voices with music, sometimes inappropriate or comic music is good for this.

Another option is to make yourself really big in the memory, as if you can become bigger and bigger until all the other people are tiny dots and you can just step over them like ants. Try doing all of these with a bad memory to see which one helps, the idea is to change something; to update it.

I like to date stamp a memory, so my mind remembers how long ago it happened, then I make it black and white and turn it into a small photograph. I stick it in an imaginary history book in my mind, and then I turn the page so the memory is not visible. I can close the book, put the book on the shelf and put more interesting thoughts on top of it.

Another more gentle way to do this ourselves, to reactivate a cue without being re-traumatised by it, is by recalling a tiny part of a memory and then doing slow breathing exercises. This allows us to only go as far as we are comfortable with and helps to change our body's reaction to the memory.

Our body as our therapist

This is where body-based therapies are again helpful to us. One easy way to create a new memory pathway in our brain is with a new movement. A new or novel movement is one the brain does not know. It might be a position we have been in before, but it isn't one our brain uses regularly, so it doesn't have a strong pathway for it.

For example, most people tend to write with one hand. There will be strong and well-used movement pathways for the hand that we normally write with. When we change hands, we feel awkward and slow because the brain's movement pathways are not used often, or we are creating new pathways to make the movement.

What kind of movement?

We need to be clear about what we want to create new pathways for. The aim of using body-based therapies is to treat ANSI (Autonomic Nervous System Imbalance) and create new movement pathways to replace ones that we don't want.

The old route that we want to bypass needs to have qualities of pain, stress, or fear attached to it. The new movements need to be pain-free, relaxing, and safe. 'Safe' means your own internal feeling of safe, not a logical judgement, or someone else's opinion of what should feel safe.

The effects of trauma can sometimes result in restricting our body movement to the bare minimum of walking, sitting, and lying down. Gentle stretches that mobilise the joints of the body, while breathing slowly and deliberately, tell the body that it is safe to move now.

All of these criteria need to be in place for the new pathway to be chosen over the old route. Remember, we want to produce a *better* route; a short-cut that has an advantage the brain wants to use. Otherwise, the brain will simply use the old route.

In chronic pain patterns that move about, like fibromyalgia, almost anywhere can be painful, so choosing very gentle relaxing movements is useful and learning to breathe correctly is also very good. We breathe shallowly when we are tense, and we breathe more deeply when we are relaxed. (I have included a simple breathing exercise you can do in the self-help section of this book.)

For people who have experienced trauma, practising being immobile, while feeling safe and relaxed is important. Breathing exercises done in a relaxed body position are good for this.

Scary stories

Fibromyalgia is characterised by erratic moving pains all over the body, with skin sensitivity coupled with unpleasant emotions and fatigue. If you take a human having these symptoms to a doctor, the doctor may try some drugs, they may do some tests, and then they may say they don't know what the problem is.

After a while of trying different things, the doctor may diagnose fibromyalgia and tell the human that their condition is incurable. They may prescribe some strong drugs to try to alter the human's brain chemistry and the patient goes home to live like this.

This is a pretty terrifying outcome for anyone's life, but this is what all fibromyalgia sufferers are supposed to live with.

We know that an expectation of pain affects our brain's response. Our brain can moderate our reactions to painful events[2] but *fear* increases our sensitivity to pain much more than expectation does[3], which is why we need to begin to resolve your fears.

Dissociation and fear

When we feel pain, it is very easy to become afraid of our bodies. Having 'unexplained symptoms' is especially scary, and being told that 'no-one knows why the symptoms are occurring' seems to happen way too often to people with fibromyalgia, even though there are plenty of good rational, scientific explanations for all of the symptoms that people with fibromyalgia experience.

When we are in pain, our body might not seem very friendly; it stops being a safe structure to live inside. We can feel like our mind and body are not connected or that our body is doing things on its own, and we (in our minds) suffer the consequences.

We might have access to the internet, which is full of information but not so many solutions and can actually cause more anxiety.

It isn't good for our health to live in constant fear. Fear actually creates more glutamate receptors in the brain[4], so the brain cells absorb more glutamate, over-stimulating the brain.

Our nervous system simply can't deal with lots of ongoing fear and sometimes the autonomic nervous system may start to implement dissociation, a numbing effect where we don't feel the body so acutely.

Dissociation can manifest in feelings of being lost, unloved, overwhelmed, disconnected from the world, or trapped. These feelings are often experienced by the sufferers of trauma or fear, and also by people who have experienced neglect or hostility from their caregivers as a child. The autonomic nervous system remains on high-alert and monitoring the external world becomes the main activity[5].

Dissociation from our physical body means we might not take care of it as well as we ought to. We might start to use our body just to get a short-term relief from the feelings and sensations we want to avoid.

Common strategies are comfort eating, drinking alcohol, using drugs, consuming too much sugar and carbohydrates, staying up late, and using electronic devices excessively. Anything that seems to take us away from anxiety, fear, or pain.

Some people take desperate measures to deal with anxiety. When there is damage to the skin, the autonomic nervous system lowers the heart rate and triggers dissociation and the numbing of emotions. These effects are biologically wired into our nervous system. Any mutilation or cutting of the skin surface, deliberately (like self-harming, or surgery), or by accident can create this 'vasovagal' reaction, starting us along the defensive cascade of the autonomic nervous system states.

For example, self-harming is thought to trigger a *Shut-Down* state[6]. This may help to explain why some people use self-harm to relieve anxiety. Alternatively, if the person lives perpetually in a dissociative state, where nothing feels real, the pain of cutting of their skin may stimulate their nervous system into a more mobilized and *Alert* state. Fortunately, we can find healthier ways to rebalance your body and mind.

We don't need to love our bodies to look after them well, but they are the only space we have to live in. If we imagine that we are going to create a lovely garden, landscape, room, or building to relax in, we can imagine that our body *is* that space and look after it to create a safe and calm place.

Feeling differently now

In this book, I am recommending that you spend lots of time doing calming activities with your body and *listening* to it, as opposed to forgetting you have a body at all.

<u>Things you need to know:</u>

Some pain is just brain signals – it occurs without damage to the body.

The fibromyalgia state is reversible.

Reassuring ourselves

Some signals, in spite of feeling painful, are not dangerous to you.

For example, stiffness in muscles can be due to lactic acid building up after exercise – and this will happen much quicker if you have fibromyalgia. Lactic acid build-up makes your muscles feel stiff and sore for many hours after exertion. Lactic acid production during exercise is normal, and the resulting stiffness and discomfort will not harm you.

Pins and needles indicate the nerves have been triggered by sensations. The nerves in our skin have also been shown to produce spontaneous signalling[7]. They can share this information to other nerves in the surrounding area, which activates the neighbouring nerves, and may contribute to sore places that seem to move about and the wandering stabbing pains that are often felt.

Brain fog can be caused by high levels of glutamate, which will clear once inflammation is resolved and your system calms down.

Unless you already had rheumatoid arthritis or a specific joint disease, then the fibromyalgia pains in your joints or muscles will not damage you or leave any lasting problems.

Stabbing-like feelings of pain that move about in the body are not caused by anything bad happening. Your brain is just convinced that it needs to tell you to be careful.

Research has shown that increases in glutamate in the brain (in the insular cortex) causes a re-organisation of the nerves in the skin (which the brain interprets as pain) but there is no damage to the brain itself [8]. This reorganisation of nerves is not permanent and can return to normal function.

Your brain is simply confused by multiple signals and is producing pain as a response.

However, all pain signals are the same. Pain signals coming from the brain in response from real damage like a broken leg or a kidney stone are the same kind of pain signals that are produced in fibromyalgia. Just because the brain is possibly creating pain signals inappropriately does not change the way these signals feel.

I want to reduce your fear and I need you to know that the pain you are feeling is *not* related to damage or a disease in your body.

The symptoms of fibromyalgia do *not* lead to disability or shorten life expectancy[9].

Normally, if we feel lots of pain it would indicate that there is lots of damage to the body but in this case it is not true. We have seen clients where their pain just stopped, proving that the body can switch off the pain very rapidly. I want to let you know that your fear of what is happening inside your body is normal, so that you can relax *with* the signals happening.

I intend that when you use the vagal toning acupressure system (VTA), reduce inflammation with your diet, and relax with slow breathing, your pain will reduce. I hope that the science in this book will reassure you that fibromyalgia is a real condition with real causes, and therefore we can reverse it. With less pain and more energy, you can start to feel the benefits and continue to find things that will help you.

14

WHAT CAN I DO NOW TO GET BETTER?

I have talked a lot about brain inflammation, and the chemical imbalance causing pain messages to become amplified or muddled. Brain inflammation might sound quite serious but, when we look at the suggested causes for it, we can see that they are nearly all under our control.

Reasons for increased inflammation[1] include:

An inflammatory diet that promotes gut permeability and changes to the microbiota (including poor-quality fats, high sugar, alcohol, and processed foods).

Obesity and a high BMI are associated with increased levels of inflammation chemicals (such as IL-6) in humans.

Psychosocial stress, particularly early life stress or trauma.

Other lifestyle factors such as smoking and a lack of exercise.

We also know that studies done on mind-body therapies such as the gentle oriental movements in yoga, tai-chi and qigong show us that these exercises can reduce inflammation in the body after only six weeks, by showing a consistent ability to reduce pro-inflammatory gene communication[2].

When we want to choose other possible treatments to help our system, understanding HRV (heart rate variability) becomes useful. We can use it as a clinical measure of how good a treatment is to help us improve our vagal function. Treatments that improve vagal function help us to de-stress us and relax the nervous system.

Treatments to improve vagal tone and reduce inflammation

Acupuncture and vagal tone

I have designed a new system specifically to treat fibromyalgia using acupressure (no needles) so that you can do it at home. I use this system with my own clients in clinic.

There are fewer research studies on acupressure than on acupuncture, but the acupoints have the same actions whether you use a needle or an acupressure *press-seed* on them (see the tools section).

Overall, we see that acupuncture can definitely help to improve (increase) our HRV[3] [4], and a study using acupoints on the scalp showed especially good results on HRV[5].

Acupuncture has shown encouraging results using brain scanning to reduce glutamate in fibromyalgia[6]. Several experts in the field of pain and inflammation list acupuncture as a recommended treatment.

Using the VTA acupressure treatments in this book can be an appropriate tool to balance the vagus nerve and reverse an inflammatory process[7]. Acupuncture points tend to have a regulating effect, bringing body functions back into normal parameters using the body's own homeostasis (balancing) mechanisms.

Research has shown that specific acupuncture points can reduce inflammation. ST.36 (see tools for the locations) reduces the inflammation chemical TNF-a[8], and SP.6 can reduce the inflammatory chemical Interleukin-10 (IL-10)[9]. SP.6 also reduces pain sensitivity to both heat and touch. [These studies used traditional acupuncture not electro-acupuncture].

Dr. Keven Tracey, a leading scientist in the field of vagal nerve treatments, gives us a list of treatments that have all been shown to improve vagal tone, including acupuncture, meditation, relaxation training, and fish oil supplements[10].

Nutrition

Diet and HRV has been studied extensively. Good nutrition has been shown to make a big impact and to improve our HRV.

A good diet has been shown to improve (raise) our HRV[11], whereas smoking cigarettes, drinking alcohol. and eating trans-fats are bad for it and will lower people's HRV. Some types of food that have been scientifically proved to raise HRV include Omega 3 fats, live yoghurts, fish oils, and multivitamin supplements.

Eating well helps to regulate inflammation in the body and can be a calming activity. Foods that create a calm internal environment, ones that help our gut to operate easily, also help our gut to produce neurochemicals that are good for our mind.

If we eat poor quality food, we are effectively saying to our body: "I don't have time to feed you properly." This tells our autonomic nervous system that our environment is stressful and therefore potentially dangerous, whereas taking the time cook and eat well tells our body that everything is fine. It tells our body that we are in charge and that we are safe.

Breathe

Breathing exercises mobilise the diaphragm, which gently massages the gut, and they give the body cues of calm and relaxation. Breathing fully, gently and slowly, tells the body that we are safe, and that we can now be calm and fully relaxed. Breathing involves many of our core muscles, and gently moves our fascia internally.

Movement

Exercise is also proven method to increase serotonin levels and improve fibromyalgia, however most people with fibromyalgia are easily fatigued and get sore very quickly. In the resources section I have given you a link to another book about Fibromyalgia I have co-authored that talks more about Yin Yoga and nutrition, called *From Fibromyalgia to Freedom.*

Yin Yoga is very calming and relaxing (it is not like 'normal' yoga and is much less strenuous). It can be a wonderful solution for fibromyalgia, allowing you to take regular gentle exercise, without causing any muscle fatigue. Yoga is known to be calming, and the existing studies indicate that it can both regulate HRV[12] and the vagus nerve[13] [14].

I have included some simple exercises in this book to move and release the fascia and relieve stiffness.

Could other activities help too?

Activities that are social, especially movement-based ones, can be good for balancing our autonomic nervous system. Choose therapies or activities that feel attractive to you, with groups that feel supportive or led by trainers you feel safe with. There is little or no benefit in working with people if you feel continually anxious with them or they are critical.

There are many enjoyable activities you could do. I have chosen acupressure and breathing in this book, and you can do these at home, but in addition I encourage you to go and find a community of people to interact with.

Walking short distances outside is really good for you. Walk slowly and don't try and push yourself, so it is something you can do daily. Being outside is good for us, and even just seeing images of green spaces is good.

Sometimes I feel agitated instead of calm – what can I do?

Anxiety is common with fibromyalgia. When you are practising feeling calm, if you experience agitation or anxiety, then the following Quick Agitation Fixes could be useful.

Quick agitation fixes

Sigh. This is the simplest reset for your body. We sigh when we relax, and after something is stressful – sighing tells your system 'it's ok now'.

Humming and chanting. Both of these are good resets for the autonomic nervous system. The vibration frequency of the human voice is the frequency we listen to most easily in *Rest and Digest*. If you like chanting, then pick a chant to repeat. If you prefer to hum then you can hum just one note, or a tune, whatever you feel like. People can often remember Christmas carols or hymns to hum.

Dancing. Most music is also calming, both slow or fast beat music. Coordinating our movement to music is a relaxing activity and listening to music is a social human activity we tend to do in groups when we are safe. Avoid really low frequency music, and instead choose upbeat, gentle, or fun types of music.

Singing along with other people singing is also really good for us. If you choose music with words, be sure to choose music with lyrics that are hopeful or loving (I would avoid music lyrics that are depressive or lack hope).

Affirmations. Speaking to ourselves, and therefore giving our brain positive instructions, is a useful thing to do. Focus on telling your body 'everything is ok now'.

Saying it out loud can help: *"Now I am safe and well, I can feel completely calm and relaxed here."*

[All instructions must be in the positive; something you *can* do. They can't include negatives like 'mustn't', or something to avoid, or *not*-do.]

Cooking and preparing food can also be a relaxing activity. You could amuse yourself by listening to comedy shows on the radio or have an audio book on in the kitchen so that cooking will become an enjoyable part of your day. Thinking about the smells of the food and how it feels to prepare food (like chopping different vegetables) are good opportunities to practise our inside awareness (interoception).

Smile. In the beginning of the *Alert* states, the body doesn't actually know if you are fearful or excited. The two states are identical, except that when we are excited and having fun, we smile. To fool your autonomic nervous system that you are excited (not anxious) try relaxing your forehead muscles and smile.

Once you feel that any agitation or anxiety is eased then you can return to your calming practices using the VTA acupressure or breathing exercises.

Returning to the affects of trauma, or overwhelming stress, we might need to move our nervous system from a *Shut-Down* state into *Rest and Digest,* and this means we pass through *Fright-or-Fight* feelings. This can feel like we are moving temporarily from a relatively quiet place into an energised and possibly anxious place.

Psychotherapists using the poly-vagal theory to help clients recover from trauma make some useful observations about how we can learn to retrain the nervous system and make these transitions[15].

To move from the *Shut-Down* state, back to feeling safe, we will have to move down through the *Fright-or-Fight* state, to get to our calm and safe, *Rest and Digest* feelings. With practice our nervous system can learn to do this progression quicker and quicker so eventually the movement is unnoticeable.

When you first start to show your body how to feel safe, you might experience feelings of anxiety, or you might feel edgy, or that you can't sit quietly. This is normal as your body energy actually increases – up from the *Shut-Down* state and into a *Fright-or-Fight* state. Your body is getting you ready for action. Stay with the process and breathe through the energised place. You might find you shake or feel wobbly as adrenaline moves in your system. This is ok and you might find walking around, dancing to some upbeat music, or jumping up and down can help to use that energy.

If it feels like it's too much you can always go back to where you were before; that's fine too. You can try it in stages.

If you prefer, you can also find a therapist (they may advertise that they work with trauma and the body) to help you work through this stage and help you to get used to coming up and down out of the mobilised states.

Using the quick agitation fixes listed above can help you move through a *Flight or Fight* state and into *Rest and Digest*. You might also like to say to yourself things like, '*I am safe now. Everything is ok here now. I am ok to relax now.*' Your unconscious and preconscious brain can hear you, whether you are speaking out loud or just silently in your head. Just thinking of safety is useful.

Depression caused by ACEs, trauma, or stress

One of the feelings associated with a *Shut-Down* state is depression. In this state the body has given up, the environment is too challenging, and so in desperation the autonomic nervous system has gone into the '*Shut-Down-and-hope-the-problem-goes-away*' mode.

Normally, if we are challenged, the body puts up a fight, we push back against people who are unkind, we avoid (*Flight*) from people who are scary or dangerous. We will struggle to stay afloat in water, and will recoil from loud noises or bad smells, which might indicate danger. In our normal *Alert!* and mobilised states we move ourselves out of harm's way.

The *Shut-Down* state is often triggered when we cannot move ourselves out of the way. We might have been in an accident that we didn't see coming or be a child and be unable or too frightened to get away from a situation. Long-term stress can convince the body that everything is just too overwhelming; it cannot cope with so much stress for so long.

Depression can be the result of this, and to get out of it we need to firstly make sure we are actually safe. We need to find some security.

It is not necessary to move through each state individually and we can move from *Shut-Down* to *Rest and Digest*. However, to move our body out of the *Shut-Down* state we may find we firstly move into *Fight or Flight,* which could feel like depression, anger or frustration.

You can find a diagram illustrating 'Depression from Shut-Down' at the end of Chapter Fourteen (page 211).

Finding our balance

Occasionally, people drop in and out of *Shut-Down*, moving from depression to anxiety (*Fight or Flight*), then feel overwhelmed again and give up, sinking back into depression. Understanding that *Shut-Down* is a coping mechanism, helps us to make sense of depressive states created by the body, and stops us blaming our thinking as the cause of it.

Moving from **Shut-down** to **Rest & Digest** by moving through **Fight-Fright**

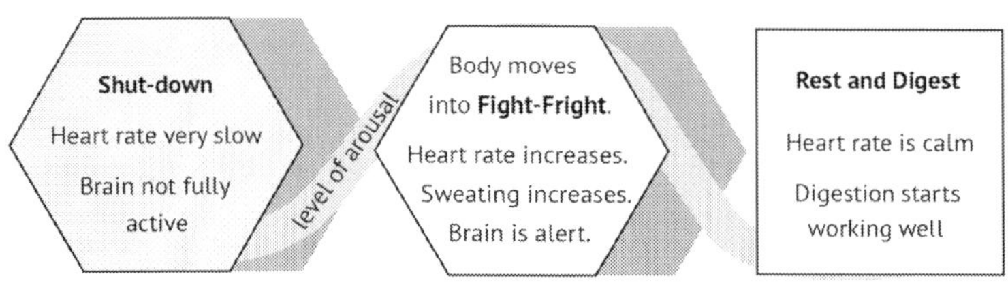

Depression has previously been blamed entirely on our thinking or on brain chemistry, and these have excluded the equally important role that the nervous system and body play in creating our 'feelings'. Once the body is calm and feels safe, the anxiety or anger can be explored and then allowed to resolve naturally, and using breath work is a key tool to help this process.

If we have experienced trauma or abuse, especially as a child, we may find that anger is triggered as we move into *Fight or Flight*. This anger and internal angst may feel frightening or vulnerable. It is likely that we could not express our own natural self-defensive anger at the time when we were a child, as it would have been dangerous or provocative to do so. We may have avowed never to be angry if we have experienced someone's rage against us. We may have associated anger with violence, and feeling anger may feel very unusual and uncomfortable for us.

What we call anger is a natural self-defence mechanism. It is a strong feeling of self-assertion designed to keep us safe and protect our personal boundaries. Conversely, violence is the invasion of someone else's physical boundaries or the use of anger to scare or intimidate another person, which as a social animal is unhealthy behaviour.

Lucia

Lucia came to see me as she was feeling fatigued and she felt flat emotionally. She said she felt no joy in her life – it was all just 'ok'. While growing up, her parents had taught her a long list of rules for living, and one of them was that she should not have strong emotions. She was supposed to be quiet and calm and not ask for much. She was given the impression that her feelings were 'too much' for other people, and this included any feelings of anger or frustration.

I suggested that all of our emotions are useful and can be used positively. This was a new idea for her. She believed anger was always negative and associated anger with intimidation, and the fear she felt when her father had yelled at her.

Lucia said that she felt as if she had been threatened as a child with an emotion (her father's anger) and she decided that she never wanted to be (or feel) like him.

But emotions are only a problem if used badly and we use them to hurt ourselves or other people.

Initially, allowing herself to experience the positive aspects of the feeling of anger, like self-assertion and setting boundaries, felt alien to Lucia. They felt like overwhelming and imposing emotions. However, when used compassionately (respecting both herself and others) she found she was able to slowly expand her emotional range.

Lucie started to realise that she actually felt angry inside because she had never been encouraged to follow her own dreams in life. She started to use this feeling as motivation to make changes, rather than just criticise herself for feeling unsatisfied.

Depression can sometimes be created by bottling up our natural energy for life but we will have *un*consciously learnt to do this, usually in order to keep ourself safe, at some time in our lives.

We can use the energy within *Fight or Flight* to reaffirm our self and our right to be here, just as we are. Anger is a natural part of our life force, and can be used for good and to make positive changes. Anger is really a kind of motivating energy within us that is created by the challenges we experience. Think of it as motivation, spurring you on to do something good for yourself and others.

How to save a life

Sometimes in *Shut-Down* we let ourselves act as if we are helpless; we say that we can't be bothered to look after ourselves or invent excuses because we don't care enough to look after ourselves, or we would like someone else to look after us, especially when we don't feel well.

As adults we know that our actions have consequences and that *we* have to look after ourselves now. We know that poor lifestyle choices can result in bad health, which can make us unhappy. Even if we were parented badly and had poor role models, as adults we can now choose a new role model.

Management takeover

You, or someone you know, may have experienced bad management in a company that you have worked for, and thought that it should be done differently. You can imagine that you are now that managing director; *you* are the MD running the organisation that is your body. You are in charge of this body organisation, and maybe you haven't really done everything you can to help it yet, but now is a great time to take a look at the direction you would like to lead it. How would you *like* to be living?

And what's the first thing that needs to happen in order to make this a reality?

Feeling motivated

If you are reading this book, then you are clearly motivated to make a change towards feeling better. The *first* change that people make might seem small but, once they feel the benefits, it strengthens their motivation to continue and make more changes. I'm reminding you of all of this because a feeling of helplessness is commonly part of all chronic pain patterns... and you need to actively resist it!

Feeling helpless and surrendering are part of a *Shut-Down* state. They indicate that our autonomic nervous system has given up fighting and now just hopes the predator or problem goes away.

Personally, I'm not keen on metaphors that describe being healthy as a 'fight' or a 'war' with disease. Our body is not against us; it isn't an enemy. Our body is simply trying to keep us safe! So, we need to work *with* our body to feel balanced and energised.

Being healthy feels good – much better than the cheap and short-term 'feel goods' from junk foods or bad living. Healthy choices are an investment we make together for our futures. You have everything to lose if not.

A new diet of calm

To create a calm mental environment and reduce your stress, avoid spending time on social media feeds that use 'outrage' to get your attention. This is a common tactic online, but it is not relaxing for your nervous system.

Similarly, you might find that it helps to avoid TV news stations with lots of graphic images of disasters and violence. Instead you could keep up to date by reading a newspaper or listening to the radio if that is better for you.

You can think about your nervous system as a kind of digestive system and consider what you are putting into it. Ultimately, *you* are responsible for what goes on in your mind and what you spend time thinking about. Self-critical thoughts are rarely constructive. Learn to distract yourself with kind thoughts, nice memories, or meditate. Make positive plans and think about how you can make them happen. There are many smartphone apps that can help you. Your autonomic nervous system responds to brain function and it responds to the *kinds* of thoughts that you are having.

If you practise making time to look after your nervous system, it can learn that coming out of a *Shut-Down* or *Alert* state and into *Rest and Digest* is a good idea because the environment you are creating is relaxing and feels safe.

In therapy

Whether you could benefit from a talking therapy is a question that really only you can answer, but if you have suffered personally from, or witnessed, trauma, violence, or abuse then you may find it helpful to have some talking therapy. Sometimes we know we need therapy but don't feel ready yet; that is fine. You will know if therapy feels like a next step for you.

Other types of therapy like EMDR (Eye Movement Desensitization and Reprocessing) and IEMT (Integral Eye Movement Therapy) are both good options for trauma and PTSD. Eye movement therapies show us that certain eye positions are connected to traumatic memories. The therapist does simple exercises with you to replace these eye movement triggers (neurotags) with better new ones. These techniques can offer fast results.

Inside our body awareness

Focusing our attention on our internal feelings uses our sense of interoception. And, in turn, using this has a positive effect on our emotional feelings because these two kinds of perceptions are linked in the brain [16]. By consciously changing our focus inwards, we help to tell our nervous system, *'It's ok now, and I can relax'*.

For instance, being still and safe can help to re-pattern the brain, and simple breathing exercises can be an excellent tool to help you achieve this experience.

Allowing your body to be still *and relaxed* allows you to experience an immobilised state *without* fear. The respected trauma expert, Dr. Kolk, emphasises how useful feeling safe and relaxed is to help our brain and nervous system change its pattern[17]. You may already be spending lots of time doing very little, because you feel fatigued, so adding some conscious slower breaths to calm the mind is a good place to start.

Exercise in general helps the brain reverse the effects of aging on the brain, especially the brain's response to inflammation. Taking some exercise regularly is really helpful for your brain to recover its chemical balance[18]. However, fibromyalgia causes fatigue that is probably caused by the alterations to the oxygen uptake mechanisms in the muscles that have been observed in many fibromyalgia studies. Take it slow and steady to get around this problem.

Start to recode the neurotags that are connecting your body to pain. Break the old connections and create new healthy ones. You'll also improve your sense of agency and gain a feeling of ownership of your body. New movements are useful, because they don't have neurotags attached to those movements.

Doing small things like using the acupressure points in this book requires very little movement, however finding the points will require you to explore your body and touch your muscles and skin in a new way. The points are designed to calm your autonomic nervous system and increase your energy.

When you use the acupoints you are looking after yourself, and you'll be making a new brain connection.

What tests do I need?

I do recommend that you see a medical doctor for screening tests to make sure that other medical conditions are not responsible for your symptoms. Some medical conditions – like Hepatitis-C, diabetes, or kidney problems – can cause damage to the nerves in the skin (peripheral neuropathy) and could underlie fibromyalgia symptoms.

B12 tests are useful too as even a relatively mild vitamin B12 deficiency can cause significant problems for nerve and brain function. B12 deficiency can cause numbness, loss of co-ordination, and pain and tingling in the hands and feet[19]. In some instances, it is necessary to have B12 injections to get levels back to normal.

- For more advice online about peripheral neuropathy you can visit The Foundation for Peripheral Neuropathy's website: foundationforpn.org

- For advice about being tested for B12 deficiency see your doctor.

[Peripheral neuropathy has been investigated as a possible *cause* of fibromyalgia but this has been discounted[20].]

Iron and fibromyalgia

Medical research shows us that generally people with fibromyalgia have low ferritin levels. Ferritin is how the body stores iron, so a low ferritin level means you are iron deficient (anaemic).

A recent European study of 100 women with fibromyalgia found that 75% of them had significantly lower levels of ferritin compared to people without fibromyalgia. How little ferritin they had was directly related to how much depression, anxiety or poor sleep they experienced[21].

Another study published in the *European Journal of Clinical Nutrition* found that having a low ferritin level (less than 50nm/ml) caused a six times increased risk of experiencing fibromyalgia![22]

What can cause a low iron level?

- Heavy menstrual bleeding can deplete our available iron and is probably the main cause of anaemia in adult women before menopause[23].
- Drinking lots of coffee, tea and alcohol can hinder us from being able to absorb iron from our food. Iron absorption may be inhibited by up to 50% by the tannic acid found in tea and coffee, and also from food additives such as phosphate found in soft drinks and food preservatives.
- Multiple pregnancies, giving blood, and having surgeries can

deplete our iron levels so much that our bodies find it hard to catch up again.

- Medicines for acid reflux (GERD) also impair iron absorption. Proton pump inhibitors (PPI) like omeprazole are well known to have this effect.
- Obesity can create anaemia, partly because obesity is a chronic inflammatory condition (see below), and partly due to an increased requirement for iron in an overweight body.
- Vegan and vegetarian diets are a known cause of anaemia. It is difficult to get enough iron from a vegetarian diet, especially if any of the factors above are also contributing.

How many people are affected by anaemia?

We might think that a westernised diet would give us enough iron, but according to NICE (National Institute for Health and Excellence) 14% of pre-menopausal women in the UK are found to be anaemic, and up to 5% of men and post-menopausal women.

Testing for anaemia

The normal test used in the NHS for anaemia is often a red blood cell count. This tells your doctor if you have enough red blood cells, which is a common way to determine if someone has enough iron. However, this test will not reveal a low ferritin level!

Iron is important and is used for many things, so our bodies always keep a stash of it as ferritin. If our ferritin level is low then there won't be enough iron for all of our body functions, even if we have enough red blood cells and haemoglobin in the cells.

One study looked at blood results for 6,993 people. Most people had the expected blood results – 130 of these people had iron tests that were 'normal' (using RBC, Hb (haemoglobin), MCV and MCH tests) but their ferritin level was low. Around one in every 53 people had a low ferritin level and were therefore anaemic, and it didn't show up using any of the other tests.[24]

Ask your physician to specifically test your ferritin levels before discounting any iron deficiencies. Ferritin should as a minimum be between 50 μg/L and 100 μg/L but some people experience disease and symptoms when ferritin drops below 100 μg/L[25].

Treatment with iron supplements needs to be continued for at least six to 12 months; it can take a long time to get the levels back up to normal. Ferrous sulphate is well absorbed but at high levels it can cause constipation, but you can go to a health store and ask for an iron chelate supplement. They are slightly more expensive, but many people find they are much easier on the stomach.

Visiting a professional nutritionist can be useful to see if other mineral deficiencies are involved with the lack of iron uptake, and to make dietary suggestions.

Iron deficiency caused by inflammatory diseases

Inflammation causes red blood cells to need replacing quicker than usual. In response to this, the body stores loads of iron as ferritin. Inflammation can cause our ferritin levels to rise, but we can still be anaemic. When older people, and those with a chronic inflammatory condition like bowel inflammation, rheumatoid arthritis, or daily alcohol consumption, become iron deficient in this way, it is called the 'anaemia of chronic disease'. There is plenty of iron stored as ferritin, but less iron is available for other uses in the body. If you have fibromyalgia and an additional inflammatory condition, ask your physician about iron supplementation.

Too much iron?

There is a genetic condition called haemochromatosis where the body stores too <u>much</u> iron as ferritin. It presents as chronic fatigue with muscle and joint aches, mood imbalances, a feeling of being unwell, and digestive discomfort, and unsurprisingly it can be mis-diagnosed as fibromyalgia!

Haemochromatosis is known as the 'Celtic disease' and it affects about one in every 200 people who has a northern European heritage. A blood test can show if the gene is present. Haemochromatosis can often go undiagnosed for many years and may only be discovered when things get worse later in life, often when the person is in their 70s.

Fortunately, it is easily treated by the person donating blood, which reduces the stored iron. Their iron levels are monitored every few months. If it is left untreated, the abnormally high levels of iron can cause liver and heart damage.

If you have northern European genetics, especially Irish heritage, and fibromyalgia symptoms I would hope that your physician has screened you for haemochromatosis.

Ask to be checked if you haven't been.

For more information about haemochromatosis see haemochromatosis.org.uk

Young people and fibromyalgia?

If you are under 21 years old then you should always seek health screening for any chronic pain or fatigue symptoms.

If you have pains in your skin or in your hands and feet, then also ask to be tested for juvenile-onset SFPN (small fiber polyneuropathy), which may present in around half of young people who have chronic pain symptoms[26]. SFPN is part of an immune dysfunction.

Prescription medications

You can carry on taking prescribed medications if they are helping you. You can add the ideas and tools from this book into your daily routine, alongside any prescriptions you take.

The biological mechanisms involved in fibromyalgia have wide ranging functions and they involve the entire central nervous system, including neurotransmitters in our brain and spinal cord. Synthetic chemicals aiming to block or alter these processes are unlikely to be able to balance all of these processes simultaneously, and the drugs might create unwanted side effects. For these reasons, in my experience the most effective way out of this disease state is to rebalance your body naturally, using a combination of non-chemical techniques. However, I also understand that sometimes drugs can be helpful as they can relieve some symptoms for us.

If you need to take prescription medications, I recommend that you *do not use* opioid medications for pain if you have, or suspect you may have, fibromyalgia. There is strong evidence that opioids are *not* effective for fibromyalgia and that they can actually exacerbate the pain. Opioids are not recommended for fibromyalgia[27] and so if you are prescribed them please seek a second opinion. If you are taking opioids at the moment, talk to your doctor about how you can come off these drugs slowly.

[Short-term use of opioids is not a problem, for instance if you are given then to use briefly after surgery. Long-term use, however is not a good idea[28]. Please discuss with your doctor or surgeon how to use opioids safely]

Depression from **Shut-Down**

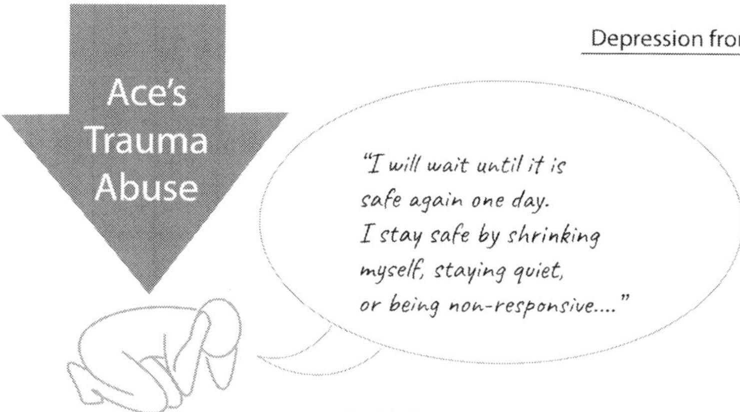

Our life force can become restricted inside a small place. It turns into frustration and can't get out ...trapped inside it turns into self-criticism.

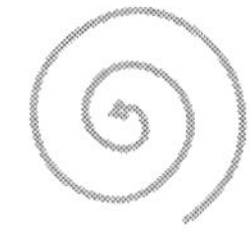

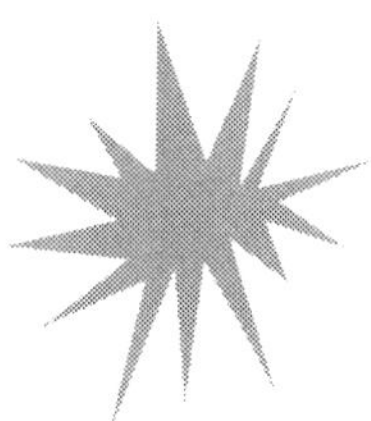

Our anger towards the person/people who hurt or neglected us, is also kept inside.

It might feel frightening to express our anger - in case it provokes them.

Maybe we don't want to ever feel like they did, and so we never allow ourselves to feel allow our own natural anger.

...but anger is part of our natural self-protection and is part of the **Flight or Fight** state

To move from **Shut-Down** depressed feelings, and through the **Flight & Fight** state, you can say to yourself;

'I am alive, and I am safe now! I can feel and I know that I am angry about what happened to me ...but I am not like them. I can use this energy for good. I can be bigger, I can be healthy, and I can achieve good things in my life.

If there is ever a time in my life when I need this protection again, I know that I could choose to assume the **shut-down** state temporarily, in order to stay safe. In my normal life I can now use self-assertion.'

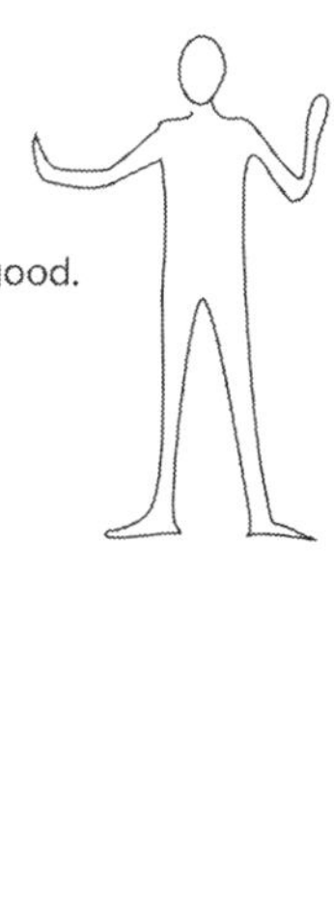

15

TAKING CONTROL OF FIBROMYALGIA

We have travelled though many ideas in this book, and I hope you can now see that there are several possible ways in which fibromyalgia can develop and be treated. I hope this information will help to show you more about the routes you can take going forward, put you back in control, and reduce your fear of the condition.

Fibromyalgia is emerging as the poster child for central sensitisation or 'centralised' pain. Brain chemistry gives us the medical proof that this is a physical condition. Even our brain function can be changed during fibromyalgia and this can be seen on MRIs, but we are also seeing people recover from and reverse fibromyalgia. This condition is not fixed or permanent – it can be changed and improved.

I hope that I have shown you that there are several possible causes for fibromyalgia and that it might require a combination of these to trigger a fibromyalgia or centralised pain state to be created:

- You may be eating food that your gut doesn't like. Gut inflammation causes permeability in the gut wall and disturbance in the microbiota. These can create warning messages in the brain or can directly increase inflammation in the brain.

- If you have experienced chronic stress, your nervous system might always be in an *Alert!* state, and it might have developed something akin to an allergic response to your environment.
- If you have experienced prolonged stress, trauma, or fear then your autonomic nervous system may have gone into a *Shut-Down* state. The resulting cognitive numbing and gut-suppression can leave the body unable to regulate the brain chemistry.
- Repeated pain experiences may have created inaccurate pain mapping in your brain, allowing normal sensations to be interpreted as dangerous.
- Inflammation from diet or lifestyle may be causing pain mapping to become disordered and increase pain sensitivity.
- Childhood adversity and traumatic events could have left your body maps more susceptible to getting blurry.

Whatever the original causes of the fibromyalgia, your body now needs *your help* to regulate itself. This is the key to the door that leads out of this state.

Your brain and your autonomic nervous system can learn and be trained[1].

Neural routes become habitual when used regularly.

I am not the only person to be proposing that fibromyalgia is a whole body, system-wide response to the environment. Scientists have already proposed that this is true[2], but new information is sometimes slow to be shared amongst the medical profession.

By taking a wider perspective, we begin to uncover mechanisms in the body that can create the fibromyalgia state. By including our emotions, past experiences, diet, and lifestyle, and adding natural treatments to improve our health, we can widen our approach to treating fibromyalgia. Understanding our biology helps us to see why we could have developed fibromyalgia, and how we can reverse it again ourselves.

This book is called *Taking Control of Fibromyalgia* for a really important reason. There are no effective 'cures' for fibromyalgia in medicine, no quick fix that will take you back to feeling healthy but you *can* be healthy and pain free again.

The more often you give your body a safe and healthy environment to live in, with good food and appropriate exercise, the easier it will be for new neural pathways to form and to resolve pain.

The path back to health is a process... not a pill.

Allow yourself to really use the knowledge in this book and keep it as a guide for you to navigate with. Because you have already learned so much about pain, you might now find that the tools I've suggested can help you to find that healthy and pain-free place to live in. As soon as you start seeing the opportunities to apply this new knowledge, you'll be able to do things differently and change will happen.

I believe you can find a route out of fibromyalgia pain, and that you can feel healthy and live well. Use the tools in this book, practise with them regularly. In particular:

- The acupressure points in this book are chosen specifically for their balancing effects on the vagus and cranial nerves in order to regulate the signals from the body to the brain. They are chosen to clear the body of brain pain and to regulate brain inflammation.
- Simple breathing exercises can give calming signals to the

body. They can be used anywhere, without anyone else knowing.
- Good-quality food can regulate your gut, reducing inflammation, helping your brain work better, and give you more energy.

Fibromyalgia flare ups

'Flare ups' is the name for the periods of time when fibromyalgia symptoms get worse. Common triggers for these episodes can be food and stress but also the weather. Food related flare ups are easy to understand and stress makes sense, given what we know about the nervous system and pain, but what's going on with the weather? So many people with fibromyalgia really dread rainy cold weather because they know they are going to feel really sore, their pain will be much worse, and their body will feel tight, stiff, and heavy.

Western science has little information to help us to understand this fibromyalgia phenomenon. However, as an acupuncturist I know that acupuncture theory has many tools to adjust how warm or cool our body feels, and to help us with the effects of weather and climate on the body.

Flare ups are often worse in dampness and cold and improve with warm dry weather. I have found in clinic that using herbal candles is a very useful treatment during these 'fibro-flare-ups'.

Using herbal candles as a treatment is even older than acupuncture. The candles or 'sticks' are made of dried herbs rolled into tubes and then lit. The smouldering herbs are used to warm the surface of the skin. This relaxing treatment is still used in Asia, where it is called moxibustion or 'moxa', and is very popular. Traditional acupuncturists also use these treatments during an acupuncture treatment, often to warm and relax tight muscles and relieve menstrual pain problems.

The particular herb that is used is a type of mugwort (Artimisia argyi) which has analgesic (pain relieving) effects and has been used by people for centuries.

The Roman troops are known to have put mugwort leaves in their boots to relieve foot pain. Modern herbalists remind us that mugwort can be used topically as a belly oil which can be rubbed externally over the womb and ovaries to relieve cramps, and that the famed 16th century herbalist Culpeper called mugwort a 'speedy and certain help for sciatica'[3].

Burning the herb releases lots of heat and it also produces a mild but particular infra-red spectrum that gently penetrates the skin when the candle is held near it. The feeling is very comforting, and I often have clients specifically request the herbal candles.

One recent study showed an improvement in ulcerative colitis, and positive changes in the gut microbiota, from using the herbal candles close to an important acupoint that affects the digestion (known as ST.36[4].

How to use herbal candles (Fibro Flare Sticks)

I have been asked by so many people where and how to get hold of the 'moxa' sticks that I use in my clinic. So, I have created a series of 'Fibro Flare kits'. They are available from my website and include a good-quality, smokeless, herbal candle and a set of instructions on how and where to use them.

I recommend you use the herbal candles during a flare up for 10–20 minutes a day. Hold the candles near your skin so that it is pleasantly warm but not too hot. You can use them on your legs, from the knees down to your feet, and on your neck and shoulders, gently moving the candles so no one place gets too hot (you will need someone to help to do your neck and shoulders safely). The gentle infrared heat can help your body to respond to damp weather differently.

"The secret of life, though, is to fall seven times and to get up eight times."

— Paulo Coelho, *The Alchemist*

Looking forward

When I was thinking about how I would describe what recovering from fibromyalgia is like, the best analogy I could come up with was: it is like learning to learn to ride a bicycle, but in a world where bicycles are unknown or rarely seen. If you had never seen a bicycle before then, watching someone ride one for the very first time, it might appear to be a really difficult thing to learn to do.

But because we see bicycles every day, we know that with practice it is possible for anyone to learn to ride a bicycle. We know that, during our first attempts, we will probably spend most of our time searching for our balance and mostly missing it. We will shift our focus in one direction, find a balanced place for a moment, but then wobble too far and have to put a foot down. We have to keep looking for that perfectly balanced place. Each time we get on the bicycle, we find our balance more easily and spend more time there. Eventually, we feel more confident because we know what we are aiming for and that we can adjust ourselves to stay on track.

As we continue practicing, we start to feel the freedom and the movement of riding the bicycle. We might still have some wobbles now and again, but we are on our way. Our confidence grows. We know all of this is possible and that it takes a little time, even if we have never ridden a bicycle ourselves, because we have seen it done by millions of people all over the world.

This is a really similar process to the one we go through when we are learning to find balance inside our bodies. To begin with, we don't know the feeling we are aiming for, but then we start to get a sense of it. We start to realise what being balanced feels like and how to correct things when we get off balance. Day by day, we spend more time in the balanced place and we can experience feeling well.

Balance is something we can only discover through moving.

Losing our balance is the only way to learn what balance feels like, and the only way to learn how to easily find it again.

When I studied martial arts, they taught us that we only know when we are balanced *because* we lose it, and the process of losing our balance and finding it again is the process of understanding what being balanced feels like. The process of losing our balance and re-finding it teaches us how to make these adjustments smoothly and more easily.

Balance in the body is not a static place; it is exactly like being on a bicycle.

We are always adjusting our weight to stay upright. This is also true of standing still on flat ground. We are not completely still; we sway very slightly. You can try this yourself:

Stand with your shoulders hip-width apart and with your head level, eyes on the horizon. Notice how your body moves, making tiny adjustments, to stay balanced. This is completely normal. Keep your body upright and just lean very slightly forward and then slightly backwards. Somewhere in the middle of these two positions, you can find a balanced place for your weight. It is also the easiest place to stand. It requires the least effort to stand upright here.

Chronic pain is something human society needs to master, and it is currently a glaring hole in our amazing medical abilities, probably because it does not respond well to the favoured medical interventions of drugs and surgery.

In the late 1800's in the UK you could go to a quiet street in a town and find determined individuals attempting to learn to ride bicycles, much like people do on skateboards today. People would find it amusing to go and watch their efforts. A Scottish newspaper in 1896 notes that 'the agonising efforts to sit on a bicycle form a spectacle worth a visit'[5].

Cycling academies run by professors also began to appear, often in large halls. People paid around £30, or monthly subscriptions, to be given an indoor lesson on a hired bicycle. Someone ran around the hall with them, holding them up and helping them acquire the skill of staying on board.

Cyclists were endlessly criticised and often ridiculed, but for many women learning to cycle allowed them a new freedom. In 1895, a female cyclist wrote in a letter to a newspaper: 'We have never yet experienced such exhilarating enthusiasm... What once was impossible has become possible, and distance is no longer the barrier to the refreshment of country life.'

Pain science is at a similar place to these early days of cycling. The pain revolution has begun and just like the early cyclists, finding their balance on two wheels in order to experience freedom, you too can start finding your inner balance in order to experience freedom from pain and fatigue.

You can become the person who can ride a bicycle in a land where almost no one knows how to. Every person who takes the route back to health helps to prove it is possible. Your recovery will help other people as well as yourself. You can now follow a route back to health and become an inspiration to others. Too many people with fibromyalgia have been told that they are simply stuck there. I know this is not true. This book is a map for a route out of that place and back to health.

I hope that having a better understanding of what might be causing fibromyalgia to occur in the first place will inspire you to see how it can be reversed. This treatment plan is a recipe that can help take your body back to a healthy, energised, and calm place.

I really hope this book is useful for you, and that the tools in the following section will help to free you from pain. I want you to take your life and energy back, so that you can shine again!

The next section contains tools that will help you work on all of the areas we have spoken about. Take your time exploring this part of the book.

I have given you a lot of information and one of the things we are all striving for when tackling fibromyalgia is a *quick* solution. Like learning to ride a bike, taking back control of your body is a balancing act that will take time to master.

The first part of mastering it, is to understand *how* it works. So, if you need to re-read the first half of the book and spend a little more time getting to grips with what is going on inside your body, please give yourself time to do so.

Particularly if you have skipped forward to read this section first, go back to previous chapters and let your brain know what's going on inside you. Then, when you have an understanding of what fibromyalgia is and you *believe* that there is a way forward… dive into the tools in the next section.

SELF-HELP TOOLS

TOOLS TO HELP YOU

This section of the book contains tools that will help you come out of your fibromyalgia state.

There is not a set prescription or combination; everyone is different, and I urge you to try each one of the key tools that I've listed to see what effect it has for you.

Earlier on in the book, we talked about the importance of healing our gut through food. I made some dietary suggestions and I would like you to revisit that section and start making small changes; you'll be amazed at how quickly you notice results, even from small, simple alterations to your diet. For a more detailed guide, as well as some fantastic, healing recipes, you might want to look at the nutrition section in my co-authored book *From Fibromyalgia to Freedom* or, alternatively, I have suggested some other books in the 'Resources' chapter on page 258.

For now, however, I'd simply like you to start by:

- Cooking from scratch where possible.
- Reducing sugar, caffeine, gluten, and dairy.

- Cutting down on alcohol.
- Avoiding refined oils, packaged or fried foods, and take-away foods.
- Increasing your water intake and your consumption of fresh fruit and vegetables.

Alongside these dietary changes, we can then look at practical tools that can have a huge impact and which you can use yourself, at home, without the need for a practitioner or coach.

The following tools are divided into acupressure (based on the acupuncture system I have developed to treat fibromyalgia in my clinic), breathing, and movement.

Each of them is very simple. In fact, they might even seem too simple to make a difference. But, in combination with a deeper understanding of what's going on in your body and an overall attempt to reduce stress and inflammation through diet and lifestyle changes, they can have a huge impact on the way your body feels.

ACUPRESSURE TOOLS

Acupuncture - how does it work for fibromyalgia?

In acupuncture theory there are the main channels or pathways inside the body, drawn as lines on the surface of the body (called *meridians*). Acupuncture 'points' are specific places on these meridians where we can access the acupuncture pathways underneath. These are the same acupoints we will be using for our acupressure in the next section. These acupoints have been found to have certain actions on the body when they are pressed or when a tiny acupuncture needle is inserted into the skin above them.

However, there are also much smaller, lesser known acupuncture pathways. If we think about the well-known main pathways as being a bit like motorways running between cities (between our internal organs), then the smaller roads are more like cul-de-sac roads in a housing estate. These cul-de-sac roads are just under the skin.

Imagine a housing development with only one road in and the same one to get out. If there is an influx of traffic to the area (say for an event like a festival) you could send a lot of cars to park here and really fill it up, but once it was full it would be difficult for anyone else to drive around those roads, and it would take lots of time to get the cars all out again as it would be congested.

This is a description of the fascia under our skin. If it is clogged up or matted it gives us the 'wet-suit', ' tight feeling in your body that you might feel in fibromyalgia.

Parking that congestion

I'm going to stick with the metaphor of 'roads' and traffic in the body in order to explain how acupuncture might help us without using any technical acupuncture terms.

According to acupuncture theory, the smaller roads under the skin can become blocked up, like a traffic jam with too many vehicles. Standard acupuncture treatments tend to concentrate on the main roads going between our organ systems because these main roads balance the big systems that are normally the cause of an illness[1].

For instance, if a person has stomach or digestive problems, asthma, hayfever, or tiredness, these would all be commonly treated on the main channels. However, if the small roads are all blocked up then we need to use acupoints that specifically move energy in those small roads.

The acupuncture points that helped

Ancient Chinese acupuncture texts tend to be concise and practical in outlook. However, when describing what it might feel like when there is too much energy in the cul-de-sac roads areas, they say that you will feel '*diffuse pain in the whole body*' and '*great emotional suffering*[2]'.

The acupoints that control our cul-de-sac roads are called the *Heaven* points of the neck, or the *Windows of the Sky* points. They are located around the neck and nearly all of them have 'Heaven' in their names, which in acupuncture theory means they are special and important points.

The *Windows of the Sky* are some of the acupoints that I found to be the most useful for fibromyalgia. They are less commonly used and are not often used together, so this treatment is a new way to resolve fibromyalgia.

I have called the set of points I am using to successfully treat fibromyalgia the *Vagal Toning Acupuncture System* (VTA) because it acts to calm the cranial nerves, including the vagus nerve, and calms the central nervous system. These points are all described in the next section where I show you how you can use them yourself, at home.

To make this information available to everyone, the VTA method is available as a short course for practitioners. So, if you would like to receive acupuncture treatments using this system you can ask your practitioner to familiarise themselves with VTA. See takingcontrol-fibromyalgia.co.uk for more details.

The ancient texts of Chinese medicine and acupuncture

I often get asked how old is acupuncture? One of the oldest books we have on acupuncture is the *Yellow Emperor's Classic of Internal Medicine*. This book is a collection of information that dates from around 2000 BCE, which is at about the same period as the beginning of the Roman Empire in Europe.

The ancient texts formed part of a sophisticated intellectual movement. At that time, there were superstitions about demons and ghosts causing illnesses, but the acupuncture texts advised people to take a logical understanding of health.

Instead of blaming ghosts, they asked if the patient had been standing out in the rain and become cold? Was the patient very tired or had they been eating unhealthy foods? This new theory looked at the whole person, and their environment, to see what was going wrong with their health.

The acupuncture texts were clearly written by people with a very detailed understanding of our anatomy[3], and they discovered how to adjust how our body feels. Acupuncture has survived over many centuries because it has proved to be helpful for improving aspects of our health. Over the centuries, famous physicians have clarified and added their knowledge to modernise the theory and practice, so that it stays relevant and useful.

Acupressure for fibromyalgia

In this section I am going to show you how you can use acupressure to heal yourself.

You may have already tried some acupressure or 'trigger' points, but this is a new system – specifically designed for fibromyalgia – that uses a different set of acupuncture pressure points to help resolve your symptoms.

How do I perform acupressure on myself?

There are two ways to stimulate acupressure points (acupoints) on yourself.

1. You can use small 'press seeds'. These seeds are held onto the skin with a small square of adhesive plaster tape, and they gently stimulate the acupoint. The seeds are either a vaccaria seed, which is about the size of a mustard seed, or a tiny one millimetre ion pellet or magnet.

This is the method I recommend you use because the effect is long lasting and it's very easy. You find the point and stick a seed on it. That's it.

2. Alternatively, you can stimulate the acupoints on yourself with a gentle holding pressure or make small strokes over the points with your fingers. You can control the sensation, so it is always comfortable for you.

Different kinds of acupressure 'press seeds'

As I said above, there are two kinds of press seeds. They are either made with an actual seed, or a tiny ion pellet or therapeutic magnet.

The ion pellets and magnets are gold or silver plated, and it is possible to buy these with clear adhesive so that they are very unobtrusive and quite pretty to wear. You can only see the tiny shiny magnet, which many people like if they are wearing them outside the home.

Both of these will work in the same way, however if you have pets or small children at your house I recommend you use the seed type rather than the tiny magnets, as the magnets can come loose and end up on the floor. The seeds may be safer if accidentally eaten by pets or children.

You can find press seeds for sale online and you can buy them on my website. They are commonly used in Japanese acupressure and for auricular (ear) acupressure.

You could also make your own press seeds at home using a small seed, for instance a poppy seed, and some adhesive tape designed for skin, like micro-pore tape, or the kind called 'sticking plasters' or wound plasters. If you make your own press seeds like this then only use them for a day or two, as the seed may start to irritate the skin if left too long.

Warning. Please do *not* buy 'press-tacks', which are very tiny metal *needles* on adhesive tape. These can be an infection risk and I worry where they might end up if they fall off, as they are very easily dropped and could harm children and pets if swallowed.

How does it work?

Press seed acupressure has always been very popular in Japan. The press seeds work by applying a tiny point of pressure to the skin, which in turn affects the fascia (connective tissue) beneath it, in a similar way to an acupuncture needle.

How will I feel?

I find that the effects of press seeds are gentle and steady. For instance, I might use them if I am feeling stressed and then notice a few days later that I have felt calmer, or more clear-headed. Gentle and steady change is what we want.

How to treat yourself using the fibromyalgia acupoints

When learning to locate the acupoints, it can be useful to use a biro pen or felt tip to make some measuring marks. If you are going to draw on your skin maybe experiment to find a comfortable pen, and one that washes off easily afterwards. A mirror is useful too.

To begin with, you'll have to refer to this book to find the acupoints, but as you get to know the locations you'll find each point quickly.

What do the numbers and letters for the points mean?

I might refer to a point as 'ST.36'. This code is part of the international numbering system that is used to identify acupuncture points. Each acupoint has a name and also a number. The numbers are not important for you to remember and I'm only giving you both the name and the number code for each point, so that if you want to look up the points elsewhere you can.

[See page 269 for more information about the code system and what the letters mean].

I will only use an English translation for the Chinese names.

How many acupoints are there for me to use?

There are eight body points in the fibromyalgia treatment:

- Four points on the side of your neck.
- One point at the back of your head (we massage this point as it's usually in your hair).
- One point on the side of your ribcage.
- Two points on your legs.

There are also four auricular points (points on the ear).

Do I use all of these points at once?

I recommend that you alternate between using the eight body points and the four auricular points. You could use the eight body points for your first session. Then on your second session use the auricular points.

I would start using them in their two groups for the first month, so that you can get a feel for the points and how they help you.

After using them for a while, you may find that there are some points you like using better than others. You can select the points you like best, which might be a mix of some auricular and some body points.

Do I use the points on both sides of my body?

Yes, for your treatments in the first month I recommend you use the points on both sides of your body.

After this, you might choose to alternate the points. It is possible to use half of them on one side of your body for one treatment, and then use those points on the other side of your body for the next treatment.

How long will they stay on?

The press seeds will usually stay on for two to three days, sometimes longer. Some people's skin may corrode the gold after a few days, so the seeds will have to be removed after two or three days if this is you.

I want to start now but I haven't got much time!

If you have limited time today then I recommend you start using press seeds on these three points: *Great Stream* - KID.3, *Wind Screen* - SJ.17, *People Welcome* - ST.9.

These three points will be a very good start. You will need to use the other points, but this will get your system moving towards a calmer place.

How many press seeds will I need?

I recommend you do two treatments a week: one treatment on the eight body points, and one treatment on the four auricular ear points.

Using these points, on both sides of your body, you will use 24 seeds a week.

Why do you recommend ear points too?

Studies show that using press seeds on the ears can make a useful contribution to reduce inflammation in the brain. The vagus nerve is closest to the surface of the body on the ear which may explain this effect.

A randomised control trial (the most stringent scientific trial) showed that auricular acupressure on ear points reduced the levels of neuro-inflammatory cytokines (IL-1β, IL-6, and TNF-α)[4]. I use three of the same points used in this study in my fibromyalgia prescription.

The eight body points

All of these points are for fibromyalgia, and they form a group that work together.

For each point, I have added some information about the special qualities it has, but don't worry if you don't have any of those specific symptoms. The main action of *all* of these points is to calm the nervous system.

Great Stream- KID.3 is on the inside of your ankle.

This point is calming, grounding, and it encourages the whole body to feel safe. It helps with fatigue, and with clearing the mind. It is therefore a really good starting place to begin your fibromyalgia treatment. It is easy to find.

Location

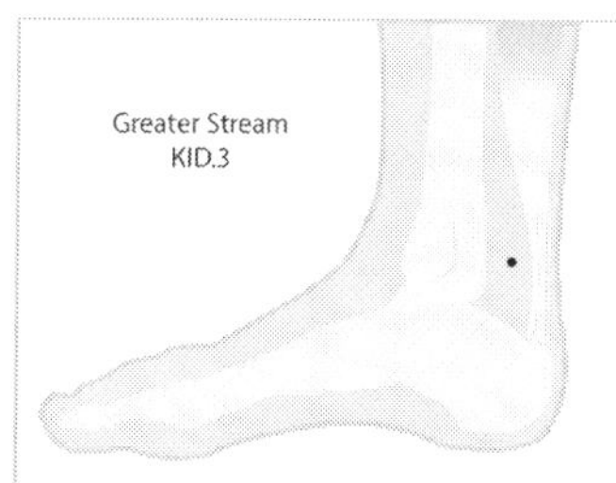

KID.3 is on the inside of your ankle, halfway between your ankle bone and your Achilles tendon (the big tendon up the back of your leg that joins your heel to your calf muscles). Find the biggest, knobbly part of your ankle joint and measure half the distance from this to the back of your leg. You will find a dip here that you can push your finger into slightly. This is the location of the point.

Wind Screen **- SJ.17**

This acupoint can be used to help to clear headaches and is very useful for TMJ pain. It can also calm the facial nerves in this area.

TMJ pain is any pain around the *temporo-mandibular joint.* It is pain you feel around your ears and the sides of your jaw. TMJ pain may also run up onto the temples of your head, or down from your ears and be around your lower jaw and face. These pains relate to the location of the facial nerves.

Location

This point is just behind your ear lobe. Feel for a dip, in the groove between your jaw and your neck muscles, just under your ear lobe, and the point is here.

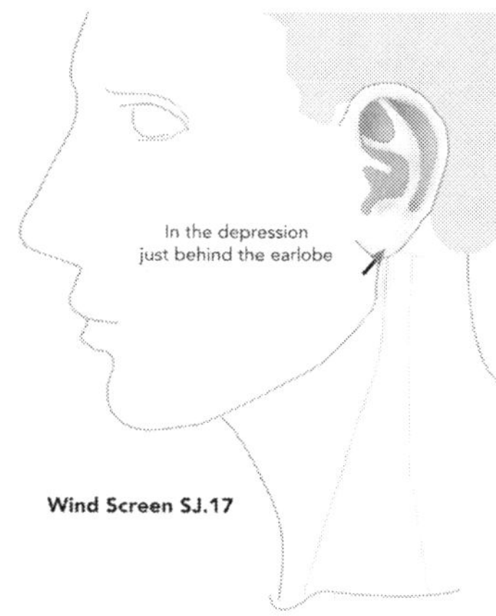

Heavenly Appearance **- SI.17**

This point calms the mind, clears the throat and chest, and helps with breathing calmly.

Location

Following the groove on the side of your neck, from just behind your ear it runs down your neck. This point is level with the corner of your jaw bone, in this groove.

[It is about an inch below the point you have just found, *Wind Screen* - SJ.17]

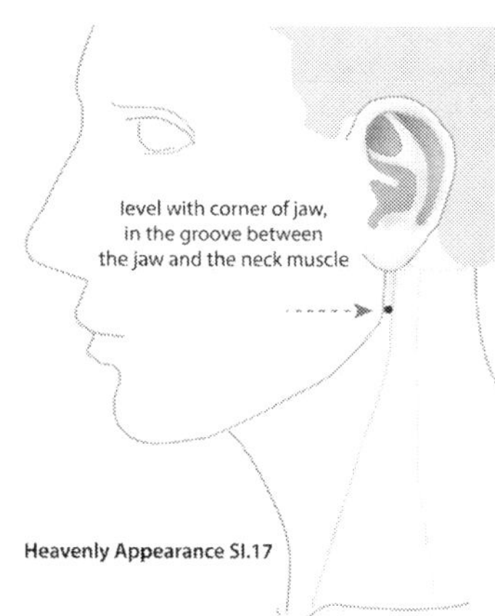

Window of Heaven **- SJ.16**

This point helps clear all of our senses – it clears dizziness and headaches, as well as neck pain and stiffness.

Location

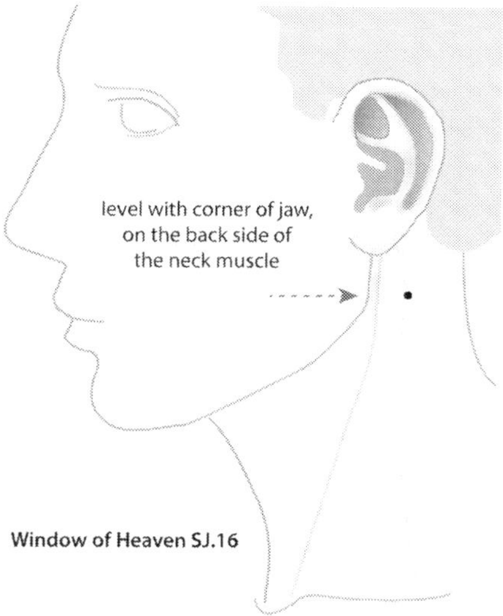

On the side of your neck, level with the corner of your jaw bone, this point is on the other side of the muscle that runs from behind your ear down your neck (slightly towards the back of your neck). That muscle is called the *sternocleidomastoid muscle* (SCM) and the point is on the posterior (back) of the SCM, level with the corner of your jaw.

If you put your middle finger just below your earlobe, on *Wind Screen* - SJ.17, then your first finger will sit pretty much in the right place to locate *Window of Heaven* - SJ.16

***People Welcome* - ST.9**

This point is on the side of your neck and it calms inflammation in the body.

It is also known as *Heaven's Five Meetings* but is most commonly called *People Welcome.*

This point is very important for fibromyalgia and it influences the vagus nerve.

Location

Start in the groove behind your ear lobe (where *Wind Screen* - SJ.17 is). Follow this groove down your neck, to the level of your Adam's apple.

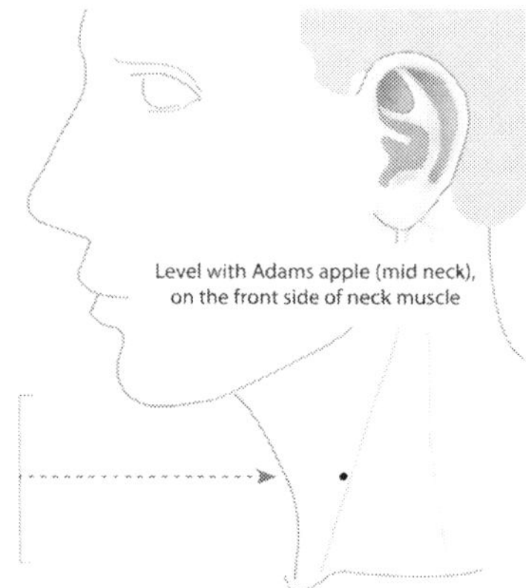

People Welcome ST.9

The most 'sticky-out' part of your neck is the Adam's apple, on the front of your neck. (The Adam's apple is also called the laryngeal prominence of the thyroid cartilage).

If you can't find your Adam's apple you can measure halfway from the base of your neck at your collar bone, up to the top of your neck under your chin.

Think of the acupoint going *backwards* towards the back of your neck (rather than sideways through your neck, from one side to the other).

Great Wrapping - SP.21

This point is on the side of your ribcage.

It is a major control point for the surface of the body. It releases a feeling of wearing a wet-suit, (feeling too big for your body), and relaxes tension around your chest. If you have read the rest of the book, this point releases those 'cul-de-sac pathways' that can get blocked.

In Chinese, the name of this point is Dai Bao. Dai means *great, big, important*. Bao means *wrapping* or *envelope*. So, Dai Bao can be translated as '*Big Envelope' or Great Wrapping.*

Location

Great Wrapping - Sp.21 is on the side of your body, half-way down your ribs, in the space between two ribs.

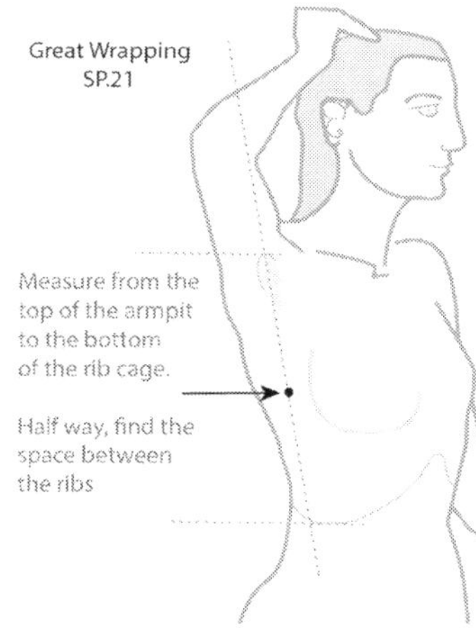

To measure which rib space to find it in, it is helpful to use a mirror or get a friend to help you.

We need to find the deepest part of your armpit, which we will use as the top measurement.

Raise your arm and feel your armpit area then keep moving upwards into your armpit until you feel like you get up to your arm. This is the deepest point in your armpit. Now, feel for the bottom edge of your ribs, at your side.

If you are using a mirror, I would mark both of these places with a felt tip or biro.

Look in the mirror and judge where is half-way between these two marks. The location of *Great Wrapping* - Sp.21 is here, in a space between two ribs.

If you find that half-way lands exactly *on top* of a bone, then press in the space that is just above or below that rib and use the rib space that is most sensitive.

Heavenly Pillar **- BL.10**

This point is on the back of the neck and influences the vagus nerve.

On most people, it is difficult to attach a press seed here as the point is usually above the hair line, so we will use a very gentle 'massage' technique on this point instead.

Location

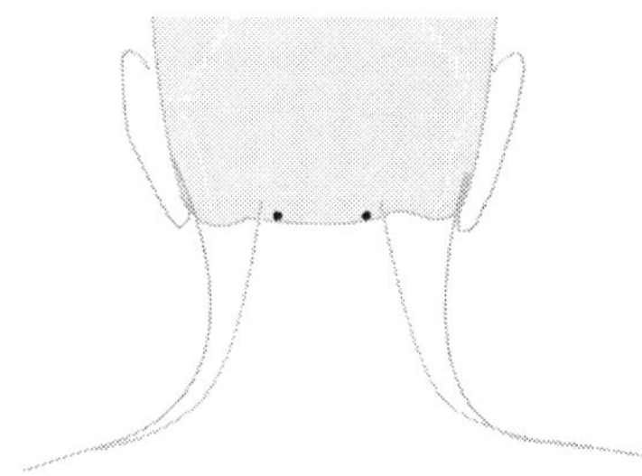

Heavenly Pillar BL.10

Place your hands at the back of your head where your skull meets your neck muscles. It is useful to move your head up and down very slowly to feel how the muscles move.

While sitting straight, firstly look downwards and you will feel there is one central muscle you can feel at the back of your skull. Then look slightly upwards. As you do so, the central muscle flattens down, and then you can feel two muscles that are now prominent at the back of your neck, about two–three centimetres apart. These two muscles are the trapezius muscles.

You are going to make gentle strokes directly over the tops of these two trapezius muscles.

Acupoint massage for Heavenly Pillar - BL.10

With your fingers make *very gentle* outwards strokes over these two muscle ridges. Each stroke starts from the centre of your neck, out over the top of the trapezius muscle, and into the dip on the other side of those muscles. Do ten of these strokes.

The strokes should be a *very light* touch. If it feels at all uncomfortable then make the touch *even lighter*!

(I do both sides at once, but you can also do them alternate sides if that is easier).

Leg Three Miles - ST.36

This point is below your knee and on the outer side of your shin bone. It is an important digestive point. It's also a wonderful point to give us a boost of energy. The name implies being able to walk for three miles after using it.

Location

Find your knee cap, which is the egg sized knobbly bit on top of your knee. Put your same-side hand on your leg just under your knee cap. Where your little finger lands is the right level to find the point. You can mark this level. Then turn your hand and put three fingers on your leg, (pointing down to your foot) so that the middle finger is on the front of your shin bone. With your hand like this the point will be next to your outer (ring) finger.

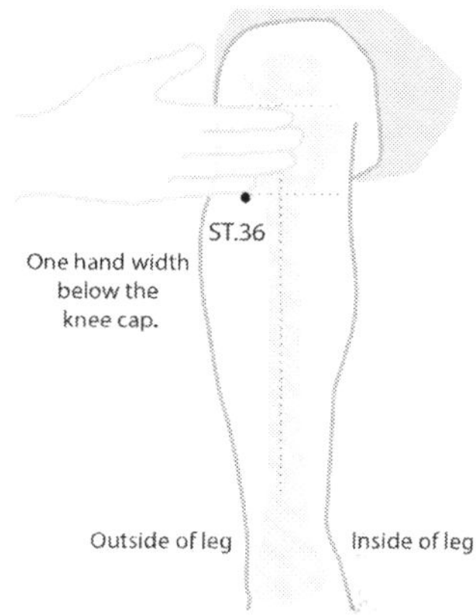

This point is on the front-facing part of the muscle, and it often feels like there is a small flat area here.

The four auricular ear points

These are the four ear points we use for fibromyalgia. These points are used to stimulate the vagus nerve and to calm the autonomic nervous system.

- Shenmen is a calming point, it is used for stress, anxiety, depression, and insomnia.
- Point Zero is to balance all brain activity and the nervous system.
- Occiput is for shock and re-balancing the nervous system, as well as for headaches.
- Thalamus is used to regulate chronic pain and sweating, and to restore tranquillity.

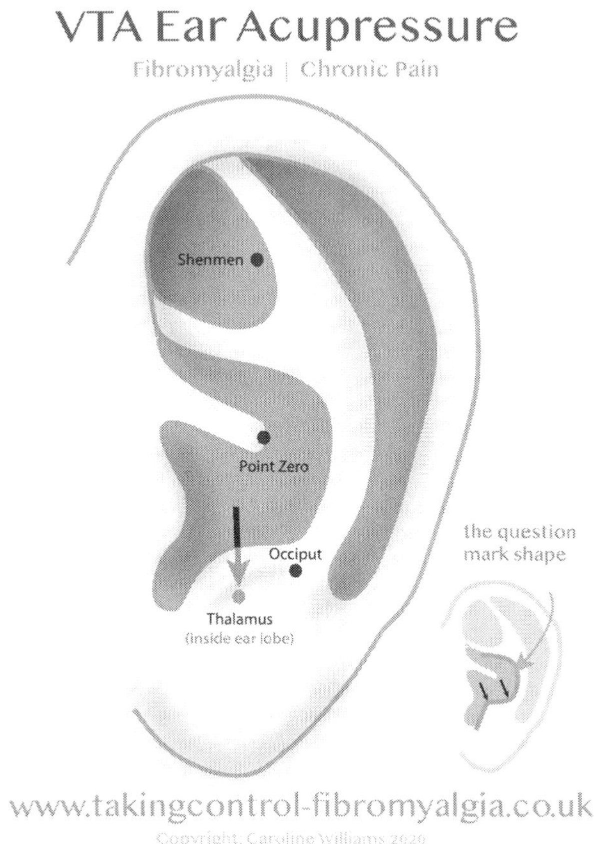

Ear point locations

Shenmen is straightforward to find using the map of the ear above.

Point Zero is where that narrow ridge turns back into a flat place, on this junction.

Occiput can be located from the map of the ear. Look for the question mark shape (see diagram) and occiput is where there is a change of direction, on the outer ear

Thalamus is tucked *inside* the ear.

Look for the question mark shape of the ear (see diagram), then from the *corner* of the question mark move over the ridge and straight down inside to the where that surface folds to become the inside of the ear. Thalamus is at this fold.

Extra body points

These are a few extra acupoints you could add to your prescription.

Great White - Sp.3

To improve digestion and to clear the mind of 'fibro-fog'.

This point helps to lift our energy.

Location

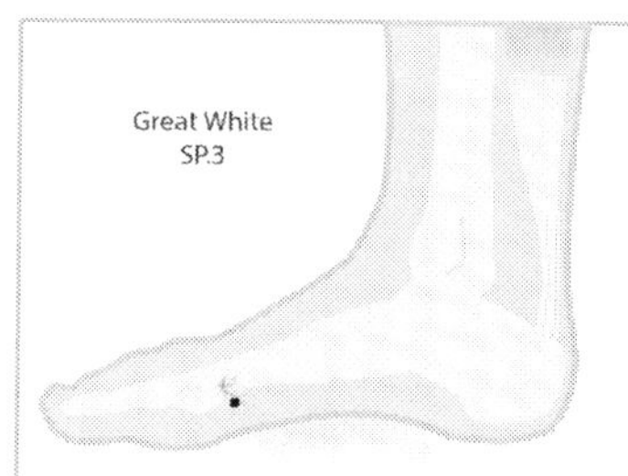

On the inner edge of your foot, feel the inside of the ball of your foot joint and then move along the side of your foot towards your ankle, into a dip.

The point is tucked in next to that bone, and just beneath the tendon that you can feel there. It feels like it is on the very edge of where your foot touches the ground.

Great Surge - LIV.3 used with *Joining Valley* - LI.4

These two points are traditionally used together as a prescription for any kind of body pain.

They will treat headaches and they are very useful 'detox' points. You can use these two points if you are reducing a medication and are experiencing any problems.

Location

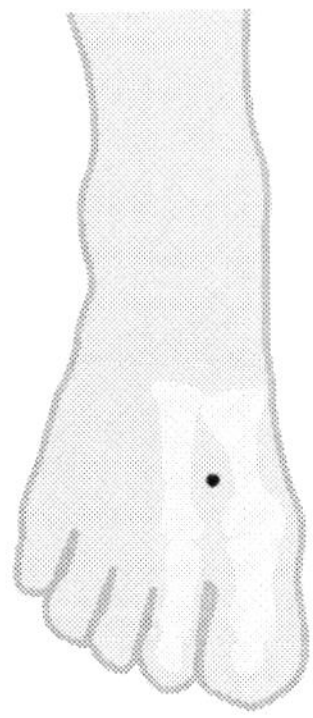

Great Surge is on the top of your foot, between your big toe and the second toe. In the dent just behind the joint of the ball of your foot.

Joining Valley is between your thumb and first finger, in the middle of the web, but a bit closer to the first finger.

Spirit Gate **- HT.7**

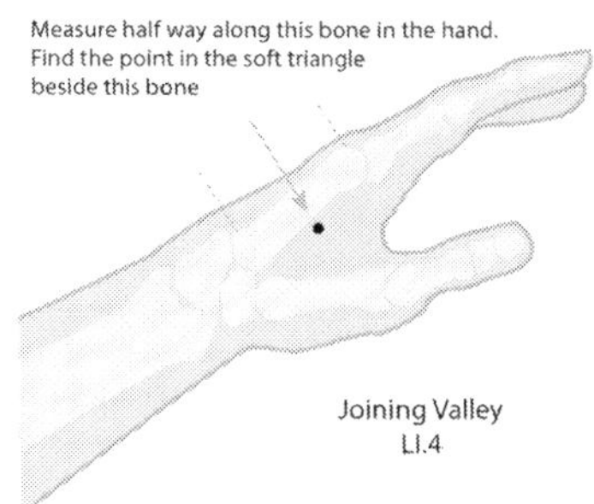

This point is used for anxiety and to improve sleep. This point is on the wrist, so it is easy to massage it if you feel anxious. You can use it with or without a press seed.

Location

At the wrist crease, on the little finger side, there is a tendon going up your arm from your hand. Feel that tendon at the crease and move to the more central side of it. The point is in this groove.

Inner Gate **- P.6**

This is another good point for sleep and anxiety. It can lift the mood and is used for when we are affected by the weather. It is also useful for treating travel sickness.

Location

This point is on the inside of the wrist. It is two fingers width, measuring from your hand crease up your inner arm, and sits between the two tendons in the middle of your wrist.

Contra-indications - when not to use these acupressure treatments

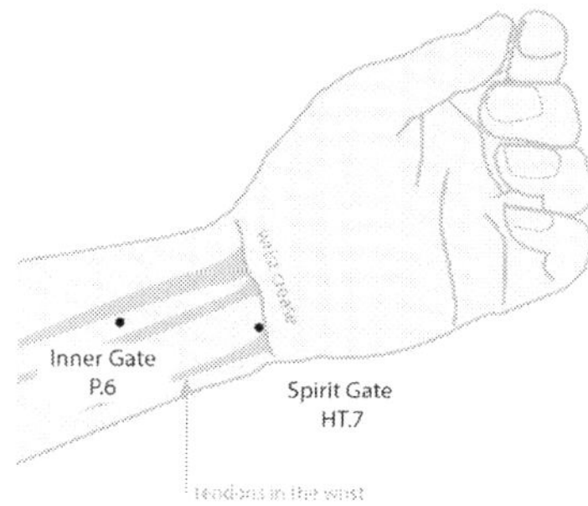

If you are pregnant, I do not recommend using these acupressure treatments.

[Three of the points listed above; *Great Stream* – Kid.3, *Leg Three Miles* – ST.36 and *Spirit Gate* – HT.7 are regularly used by acupuncturists to treat pregnant women and are generally regarded as safe to use in pregnancy].

If you have a perforated eardrum please do not use any of the ear points on that/those ear/s.

If you have diabetes or a skin condition like eczema on your ears, please be careful not to leave the seeds on too long as it could cause skin irritation or infection.

BREATHE ME

This is a simple breathing exercise for you. It asks you to gently slow your breathing rate, and to breathe out for longer than you breathe in.

Before you start anything, while you are sitting and relaxing, you can measure your natural breathing per minute. One breath in, plus one breath out, counts as 'one whole breath'. Make a note of how many whole breaths you tend to take per minute without altering anything about your breathing. This will be useful when we look at choosing a speed to breathe.

Taking slower breaths can calm the nervous system. This breathing exercise is flexible and can fit everyone:

- Sit comfortably with your back straight. Or stand with your feet at shoulder width apart.
- You are going to count to four as you breathe in, 1 - 2 - 3 - 4
- While you breathe in, stay relaxed. Your shoulders should not move upwards or be pulled up towards your ears. Your neck and shoulders can always remain relaxed.

- Once you have breathed in fully, you can pause slightly, but do not close your throat.
- If you whisper the sound 'arhhh', this is the sound you can make on your out-breath.
- Count to six (in your mind) as you breathe out, making the sound 'arrhhh'.
- The out-breath has a little push to it because of the 'arhhh' sound. This helps the out-breath air leave your lungs at a steady pace.
- Let the air leave your lungs gently, there is no need to push the last of the air out of your lungs with force.
- Once you have breathed fully out, relax and notice the place between the out-breath and the next in-breath. When it feels natural to do so, start the next in-breath.
- Continue to breathe in... pause... and breathe out... and relax ...
- The out-breath should take a little longer than the in-breath.

If you need to stop, or feel like you want to breathe normally for a while, that's absolutely fine. Just start again when you feel ready.

Even doing a few slow breaths regularly are useful. As you practise this for a few minutes every day it will get easier and slightly addictive!

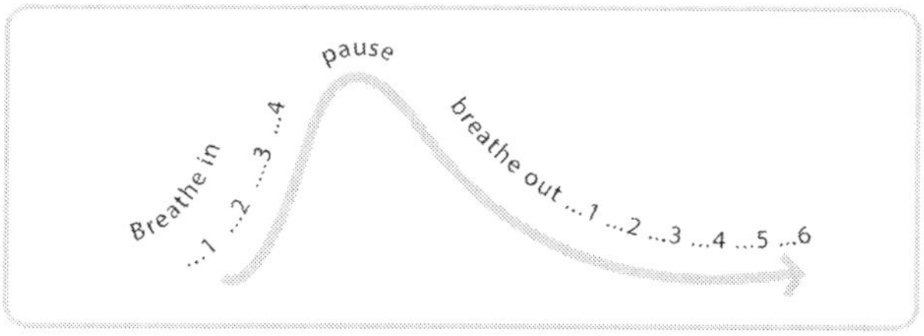

Keep the throat relaxed and open when the lungs are full, so there are no 'stops' between the in-breaths and the out-breaths.

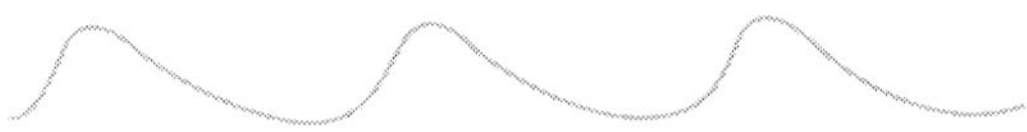

At what speed should we do breathing exercises?

The speed of breathing depends on your natural rate. For example, if your natural breathing rate is 12 whole breaths per minute, you could do ten whole breaths a minute and if that is ok, you could try nine whole breaths a minute. See what works for you. Just aim for one, or maybe two, breaths less per minute than your resting breaths.

When we breathe slowly and deliberately, we tend to breathe more deeply, so we do not need as many breaths. The pause at the top of the breath, and the relax at the end of the out-breath, can help to balance the extra air we take in.

Walking on air

If you feel at all short of air, please relax and breathe normally for a while. Always breathe when your body wants to. Do not try and hold your breath. Follow your body, not the clock.

If you feel at all dizzy, stop doing this exercise until you feel fine again. Breathing too much and too fast can make us feel dizzy. Wait a while before you try again, at a different speed, sometimes slower might help (fewer breaths per minute), but *listen* to your body.

Tools to help

We can use smartphone apps to help us. The one we recommend at our clinic is the 'Insight Timer', which is free to download from the App Store. You can use it to create a timer or find relaxing music for your session.

You can also save a 'pre-set' timer that you can design. I find having a timer that I have made for breathing makes it more fun to practise. I have a particular gong to start, with some quiet music for the timer and then another gong to finish. Even the free version of the app will record how many days you have practised. The paid-for version has lots of extra relaxation courses on it.

Born to move

You can also do this breathing while sitting, walking, or dancing very slowly. Combining this exercise with slow walking creates a really good mindful walking meditation.

You could make up some flowing movements to do with the breathing, any random gentle movements you like are great. Or you can do some gentle stretches while doing the breathing, which is also a lovely combination.

For practical ideas about how to incorporate calmness into your life, I would recommend the beautifully written and friendly guide to meditation and mindful living: *Inhale - Exhale - Repeat: A meditation handbook for every part of your day,* by Emma Mills.

EXERCISES FOR THE FASCIA

You'll be relieved to hear that the type of exercises that help our fascia don't need our muscles to work hard.

I'm going to show you some easy exercises where you swing your arms and legs gently to stretch and tone the fascia. These are surprisingly effective, they take only about ten minutes to do them all, and you will be able to do them regularly without getting problems from your fibromyalgia. They are based on principles of movement from Japanese yoga, (*Hitori-Ryoho,* which means self-healing) and influenced by *Anatomy in Motion* developed by Gary Ward.

I have a free video on my website that you can follow too at takingcontrol-fibromyalgia.co.uk

All of these movements should be relaxed and smooth. They should not feel stiff or jerky. You can guide the amount of movement, so it is comfortable for you to do.

ARMS

In these arm exercises imagine your hands are heavy, especially your little fingers.

Shaking the arms out

Shake your hands as if you are shaking water off them. It doesn't really matter which way your hands fold; the feeling is to get all of your arms moving in a steady rhythm. Feel the movement go up your arms to your shoulders.

Then slowly stop shaking, little by little until you are still again. This often gives a nice tingling feeling.

Arm swings

The feeling in these exercises is that the arm swing will start from the little fingers. The arm is relaxed and has an elastic feeling.

Do as many swings as is comfortable – eight swings in each exercise would be ideal.

Swinging arms in front of you

1. Stand with your feet shoulder width apart. Allow your knees to relax or even bend a little, just so the joint is not stiff or tense.
2. Take your arms a little way away from your body and imagine you are standing waist deep in light and fluffy snow. You are going to scoop up some snow and guide it forwards. Imagine it will land on something (or someone) who is about three metres (12 feet) away from you. Keep your arms relaxed as you swing them both forwards and bring your hands together into a scoop in front of you, ending up about the same level as your nose. Your arms will naturally bend at the elbows as they swing forwards.

3. Then allow your arms to swing back to just behind you to collect another scoop of imaginary snow.
4. Keep your shoulders relaxed. They should not rise up with your arms.

This exercise is useful for the backs of the arms and base of the neck.

Snow circles while standing

1. Stand with knees relaxed, feet shoulder width apart again.
2. This time, raise both arms in front of you to about waist level. Keep your belly button facing forwards and keep looking forwards. Both arms are going to swing around you in an arc around your left side. Stay looking forward but allow your shoulders and ribs to follow your arms. Your left arm will swing back as far as is comfortable and your right arm will wrap around your body.
3. Then allow the elastic feeling in your body to swing your ribcage and arms back to facing forwards again and continue round the other way.
4. Swing your arms gently around from one side to the other side a few times.

Keeping your head still and looking forward in this exercise will stop you from getting dizzy. Japanese yoga emphasises balance and co-ordination in all movements. This movement gently wakes up our whole spine and the lower back. Keeping your head and your belly button facing forwards, while your arms and ribcage rotate from side to side, encourages correct spinal movements in walking.

If you did this exercise while you were standing up to your waist in snow you might make a circle around you in the snow.

LEGS

For the legs, it is good to have something to hold on to or touch, in order to help with balance. A kitchen worktop is ideal, or you could use the back of a chair.

Shaking our legs out

Hold on to the worktop or chair and shake one of your feet.

Imagine that there is water on the top of your foot and that you are going to gently shake it off. Let the movement become rhythmic so the gentle shaking feeling goes from your foot and all the way up your leg. You can probably feel the muscles in your legs wobbling with the movement, which is good. The leg is relaxed. Then slow down very slowly until you come to a stop again.

Change legs and shake out the other leg.

Elephant walking

If you have a large book, it can be useful to stand on. This exercise helps to release tension in the lower and middle of our back, which can be very nice first thing in the morning.

1. Stand next to the worktop/back of chair.
2. Stand on the leg closest to the worktop, and gently swing the other leg backwards and forwards, like walking.
3. Now bend forward slightly and relax your head down, to look at the floor. Swing your leg the same way and while you are swinging the leg you can also swing your arm on the same side. Swing your arm in the opposite direction to the leg, so that your leg goes forward as your arm comes back. I like to think I am like an elephant walking.
4. Relax the swinging foot and arm as much as possible. Just let the weight of the arm and leg hang as you swing them. Relax

the neck as much as possible. The further that you bend over, the lower in your back you'll feel the movement.

5. By raising or lowering your upper body you can work on different parts of your back.
6. Change round to stand on the other foot and swing your leg and arm on the other side.
7. If you have a large book or a 'yoga brick', you can stand on the book/brick to get a little height. This helps you to relax the swinging foot a little more.

SIDE BENDS – the easy way

Most side bends ask you to bend mostly in the body, which can be hard work. This stretch is different and it repositions one of your feet, making it much easier to get a nice stretch without moving your upper body too much.

1. Stand facing the worktop/back of chair.
2. Take one leg and put it just behind your standing foot with the top of this foot facing the floor (like they do in ballet). Relax this leg, so that your knee is slightly bent. Allow your hip to drop lower on this side. This feels like your knee and bum get closer to the floor. (If this foot is not comfortable on the floor you can put a towel under it).
3. Now, bend your body over to stretch away from the side with the bent leg. Let your bent-leg hip drop down, and bend your body gently over sideways to lengthen that side of your body.
4. If that is easy, then you can raise your arm on the same side as the bent leg and stretch your arm up and slightly over as you bend sideways.
5. Change around and stretch the other side.

Using left and right instructions

Standing on your right leg, hold on to the worktop with your right hand. Relax and bend your left leg and put it behind you so that the foot is resting on the floor with the top of the foot on the floor. Drop the left hip so it feels like your left knee gets closer to the floor. Raise up your left arm and stretch gently upwards and slightly over your head as you allow your body to bend slightly to the right. Come back up to centre and change sides.

Standing on your left leg, hold on to the worktop with your left hand. Relax and bend your right leg and put it behind you so that the foot is resting on the floor with the top of the foot on the floor. Drop the right hip so it feels like your right knee gets closer to the floor. Raise up your right arm and stretch gently upwards and slightly over your head as you allow your body to bend slightly to the left.

This exercise opens up the whole side of our body and doesn't require muscular strength. Dropping the hip on the stretching side is important, as it helps to release tension in our pelvis.

You can allow your head to go over sideways with your body, and you can also try keeping it upright (eyes level) while you are stretching.

To increase the stretch, slide the bent leg foot further so your body makes a C shape, from your foot up to your arm in the air.

SLIDING PELVIS GLIDES

These pelvis glides stretch out our waist and our spine, which is useful for walking. When I say pelvis I also mean your bottom.

Standing up, raise one arm to your side (as if you were signalling to turn that way on a bicycle). Now lean your weight onto your opposite foot, and as you do so you can move your pelvis (bottom) sideways, away from your signalling arm. The signalling arm helps you to stay balanced as you take your weight in the other direction. Keep facing forwards, eyes and head level.

Using left and right instructions

If you raise your right arm out to the side, take your weight more onto your left foot, and as you do so, slide your pelvis left. Come back to the middle and this time raise your left arm out to your side, take your weight more into your right foot, and as you do so, slide your pelvis to the right side.

Check your pelvis slides over without twisting, your belly button should stay facing forwards, not off at an angle. If you are not sure, put a finger on your belly button, it will helps you to see which way your pelvis is moving.

SEATED JAW and NECK RELEASE

Sit upright on the edge of a supportive chair (something like a kitchen or office chair, not a sofa). Both feet on the floor. Eyes on the horizon.

Keeping your shoulders still, and balanced over your bottom, arch your back so your ribcage sticks out forwards and your back is hollow. Your head should stay level (not tipped back).

Check - has your chin moved? People's chins often move upward when they arch their back. Remember to keep your head and chin still as you arch your back. Your chin will need to move closer to your chest as you arch your back.

Now raise your arms, keeping your shoulders down. Raising your arms will help to arch and extend your back. If it is comfortable to do so, raise your arms so they are next to your head, palms facing forwards.

In this arched back position allow your jaw to relax, open your mouth slightly and wiggle your jaw slowly from side to side. Stretch your jaw forwards so your lower teeth are in front of the top ones.

And then lower your arms and relax, into your normal sitting position.

Now we will do the opposite posture.

Allow your back to round over. As your whole back rounds over you will find you become very short. Allow your head to jut forwards, still keeping your head level and your eyes on the horizon.

Raise your arms in front of you, this time only to shoulder level, palms facing down (as if you were going to dive forwards). In this place you can find a lovely stretch in the middle of your back and shoulders.

In this rounded back, arms forward position, again relax your jaw, open your mouth slightly and this time take your jaw slightly backwards towards your chest (leave your head where it is). Move your jaw gently to the right and to the left. Then open your mouth fully as far as is comfortable.

Then relax and sit normally.

Some people like to end this exercise by doing the arched back version again to end with.

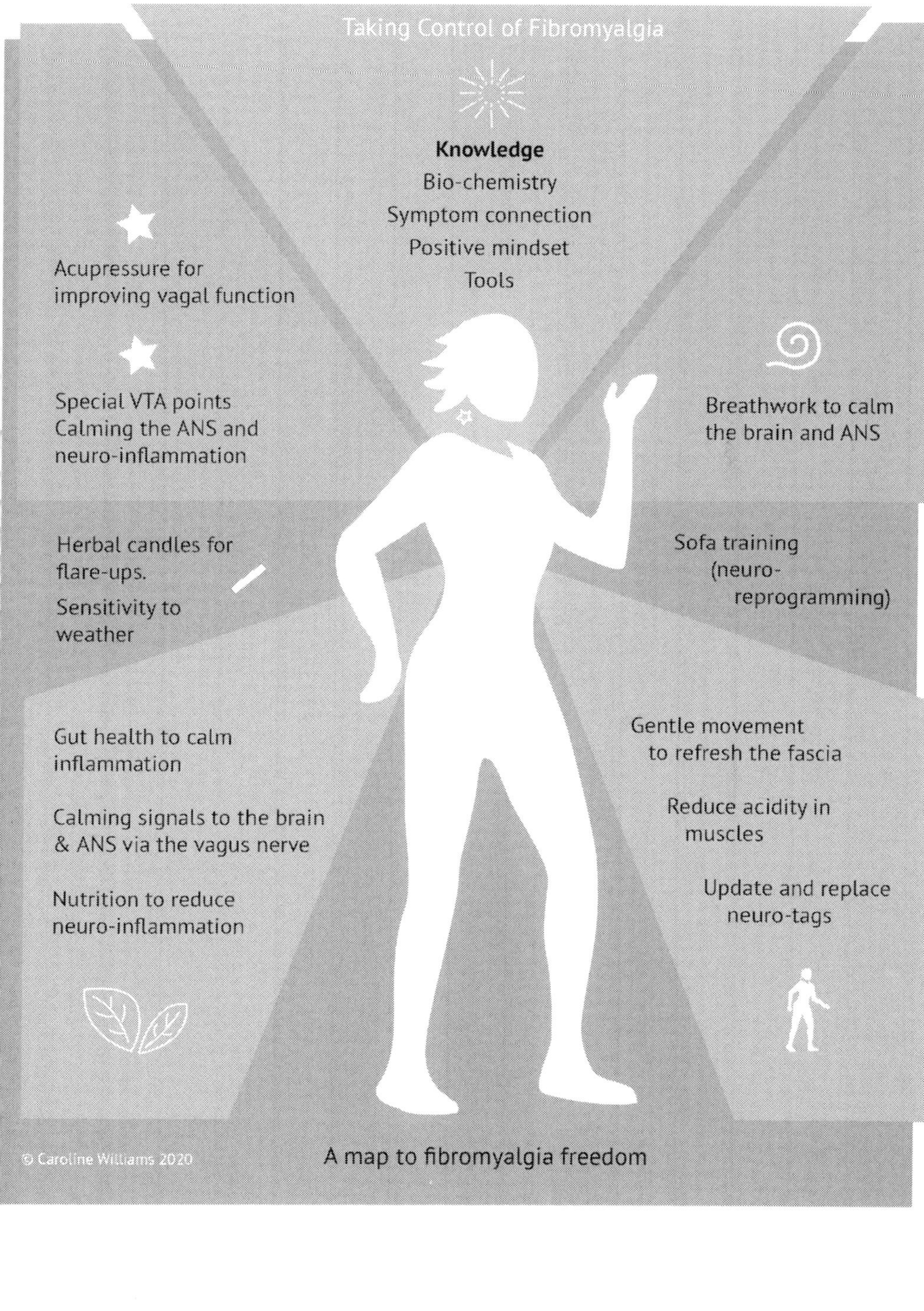

Taking Control of Fibromyalgia
Knowledge
Bio-chemistry
Symptom connection
Positive mindset
Tools
Acupressure for improving vagal function
Special VTA points Calming the ANS and neuro-inflammation
Breathwork to calm the brain and ANS
Herbal candles for flare-ups.
Sensitivity to weather
Sofa training (neuro-reprogramming)
Gut health to calm inflammation
Calming signals to the brain & ANS via the vagus nerve
Nutrition to reduce neuro-inflammation
Gentle movement to refresh the fascia
Reduce acidity in muscles
Update and replace neuro-tags
© Caroline Williams 2020
A map to fibromyalgia freedom

AUTHOR'S NOTE

This book was written because one of my best friends has fibromyalgia.

I met a fellow therapist, Clair Starr, in 2005 while we were both working from a yoga centre. We became friends, and then in 2009 we opened our own therapy clinic together. By then she was a successful corporate coach and it came as a shock to see my energetic and upbeat friend start to suffer with pain and fatigue, and even more worrying when she didn't seem to be getting over it.

When Clair's doctor diagnosed her with fibromyalgia, they told her that she would end up in wheelchair and recommended that she give up doing everything strenuous, but Clair refused to give up. With a large network of therapist friends, there was no lack of choice of therapies to try. But nothing over the years really seemed to make a difference that lasted.

The better I understood the fibromyalgia condition, the more it seemed strange that acupuncture wasn't making more of an impact. I went back to first principles, reading the classic texts, and then the scientific research. And I uncovered a different approach. The new acupuncture points I found were also over vagal nerve control areas, linking ancient wisdom to modern science.

At the same time, Clair was encouraged to write a book about everything she had found out about fibromyalgia. We knew by then that fibromyalgia responded best to a combined approach. So three of us set out to write a book, with Ellie Coston covering nutrition, Clair telling her own story and journey with yin yoga, and me writing about acupressure.

However, as I read papers on medical research, I found more and more information that was really important for fibromyalgia. I was surprised to find so much knowledge about fibromyalgia symptoms when the medical profession would have us believe that fibromyalgia is a mysterious condition!

It was a long, slow year collecting the information and writing it up. My other half was endlessly patient as his partner buried her face in a laptop day after day.

Finally, ten months later, we sent our contributions to our book editor. We had been advised to publish independently because publishing companies don't often accept group-authored books like ours. This seemed odd to me, as in any other situation getting advice from *three* professionals would be considered better than just one!

When we looked through what we'd written, it turned out that we actually had *so much* information that we had to publish it in two books! So, I returned to my laptop (more sighs from my partner) to convert my research into this book, *Taking Control of Fibromyalgia.* It was a lot of work, but I am happy knowing that you are now able to easily access all the tools we use in our clinic, and the science behind them. I want to give everyone the information they need to get well.

The book the three of us wrote together is called *From Fibromyalgia to Freedom.* It tells Clair's personal story, and it begins the path to getting well from fibromyalgia using nutrition, movement, acupressure, and other useful tips.

We are all very passionate about changing the world for fibromyalgia sufferers. I am always disappointed every time I hear of someone with fibromyalgia having their symptoms dismissed, or disbelieved, and I really hope our books will contribute to a change in attitude.

Before I say goodbye to you here, wishing you every encouragement on your fibromyalgia journey, I have a request on behalf of other fibromyalgia sufferers. If you have found the information in this book useful to you, please could you take a moment to write a review to help other people to find it too, because everyone with fibromyalgia deserves support.

Best wishes,

Caroline

You can leave your review here:
http://www.amazon.co.uk/Taking-Control-Fibromyalga-Following-Science-ebook/dp/B08DG8BWWG

RESOURCES

Heart Rate Variability (HVR)

Heart Rate Variability (HVR) several measurement apps are available on app stores. A simple one is fine. Some apps have extra information added for athletes in training schedules which you don't need to pay for.

Guided Motor Imagery

http://www.gradedmotorimagery.com

Search on YouTube for 'What is Graded Motor Imagery' for a 3.5 minute video explaining it. [https://www.youtube.com/watch?v=fWYUJscRBRw]

The Graded Motor Imagery apps are called 'Recognise' and have an orange logo. Arms and legs are divided up, so there is a Recognise-Hand, and a Recognise-Foot version.

Other online resources

The Chronic Pain and Fatigue Research Centre, University of Michigan publish useful information about fibromyalgia and you can also find videos from Dr. Daniel Clauw and his team: https://medicine.umich.edu/dept/chronic-pain-fatigue-research-center

The Foundation for Peripheral Neuropathy: https://www.foundationforpn.org/

Eye Movement Desensitization & Reprocessing: https://www.emdr.com/

Integral Eye Movement Therapy https://integraleyemovementtherapy.com

Tools for fibromyalgia

Fibro Flare kits are available from: www.takingcontrol-fibromyalgia.co.uk

Books

***'From Fibromyalgia to Freedom'* Clair Starr, Eleanor Coston, Caroline Williams.** The book I co-authored with two other therapists, including my friend Clair who is a fibromyalgia sufferer, where we take a wider look at practical lifestyle advice to restore health, and at Clair's story of recovery from fibromyalgia back to health.

'*The Body Keeps the Score*' van de Kolk. A very good book on childhood trauma and post traumatic disorder, by a highly experienced practitioner.

'*Accessing the Healing Power of the Vagus Nerve*' Stanley

Rosenberg. Chiropractic exercises you can do yourself and information about the vagus nerve.

'***Stumbling on Happiness***' **Daniel Gilbert.** An entertaining explanation of how we make decisions, and think about our future.

'***Interoception - the eighth sensory system***' **Kelly Mahler.** Easy to read with lots of simple exercises to help increase internal awareness. Could be used with children too.

'***Rip it Up***' **Richard Wiseman.** A very readable book about the psychology of acting 'as-if,' and how our behaviour and our beliefs are connected.

'***Inhale. Exhale. Repeat: A meditation handbook for every part of your day***' **Emma Mills.** A lovely guide showing us how to include meditation, calmness and mindful living into our daily life.

'Childhood Disrupted: How Your Biography Becomes Your Biology, and How You Can Heal' **Donna Jackson Nakazawa.** This book explores more fully how trauma in childhood can affect our health as adults.

'Swallow This, Serving up the Food Industry's darkest secrets' **Joanna Blythman.** If you wondered why processed food is always on a list of foods to avoid, this book is both scary and enlightening. You will never look at a packet meal the same way after reading this book.

APPENDIX

The eighteen tender points?

Previously, eighteen 'tender points' were used to diagnose fibromyalgia. If more than eleven of them were sore then the person had fibromyalgia. This method of diagnosing fibromyalgia has been discredited and is not used any more.

International Acupuncture Point Code

Each acupuncture point has a letter and number code, so for instance ST.9 is code for; stomach meridian, point number 9.

The major lines of acupuncture points on the surface of the body (main meridians) are named according to the organ system they can influence.

Most of the points on a meridian will affect the function of the organ they are named after. They *also* affect the emotions and other body functions that are associated with that organ system. For instance, the ‘liver ’ in acupuncture theory is responsible for managing stress and giving us flexible tendons, as well as ‘normal’ (western) liver functions. In acupuncture theory the meridians use capital letters to show the difference between an actual bladder, and the bladder meridian.

Meridians will also have an effect on other parts of the body that they travel through. So, the Small Intestine meridian travels over the shoulders and down the sides of the arms and we can use it to treat shoulder pain as well as gut related symptoms.

For instance: there is a bladder meridian which is abbreviated to ‘BL’.

The meridians each have a starting and ending point.

Each point on that meridian is given a number starting from one so Bl.10 is the tenth point on the bladder meridian.

All 14 of the main meridians are numbered this way. The abbreviations are:

Heart meridian = HT

Small Intestine meridian = SI

Large Intestine meridian = LI

Lung meridian = LU

Gall Bladder meridian = GB

Liver meridian = LIV

Kidney meridian = KID

Bladder meridian = BL

Ren meridian = REN

Du meridian = DU

The VTA points for fibromyalgia are numbered on these traditional meridian lines.

A NOTE ON REFERENCES

Nearly all of the research papers cited in the Endnotes section of this book are fully and freely accessible online.

REFERENCES

Losing your life to pain - and getting it back again

1. Kissin I. (2015). Scientometrics of drug discovery efforts: pain-related molecular targets. *Drug design, development and therapy, 9*, 3393–3404.

Mapping the territory

1. Butler, D. S. (2000) The Sensitive Nervous System. Noigroup Publications.

1. The chemicals between us

1. Harris, R. E., Sundgren, P. C., Craig, A. D., Kirshenbaum, E., Sen, A., Napadow, V., & Clauw, D. J. (2009). Elevated insular glutamate in fibromyalgia is associated with experimental pain. *Arthritis and rheumatism, 60*(10), 3146–3152.
2. Littlejohn, G., & Guymer, E. (2017). Modulation of NMDA Receptor Activity in . *Biomedicines, 5*(2), 15.
3. Kraal, A.Z., Arvanitis, N.R., Jaeger, A.P,. Ellingrod, V.L (2019) Could Dietary Glutamate Play a Role in Psychiatric Distress? *Neuropsychobiology*.
4. Lowy, MT., Gault, L., Yamamoto, BK.(1993) Adrenalectomy attenuates stress-induced elevations in extracellular glutamate concentrations in the hippocampus. *Journal of Neurochemistry* 1993; 61: 1957–1960.
5. Harte, S. E., Clauw, D. J., Hayes, J. M., Feldman, E. L., St Charles, I. C., & Watson, C. J. (2017). Reduced intraepidermal nerve fiber density after a sustained increase in insular glutamate: a proof-of-concept study examining the pathogenesis of small fiber pathology in fibromyalgia. *Pain reports, 2*(3), e590.
6. Mangia, S., Giove, F., & Dinuzzo, M. (2012). Metabolic pathways and activity-dependent modulation of glutamate concentration in the human brain. *Neurochemical research, 37*(11), 2554–2561.
7. Oxidative stress is an imbalance inside the body, between waste products, and the good chemicals our body uses to neutralise them. In very simple terms the body becomes toxic (imagine the health of a goldfish if you didn't ever clean the water in the tank).

   Things that can cause oxidative stress are; rancid or overheated vegetable oils (think fried food or cheap cooking oil), pesticides (some foods are more sprayed than others), plastics (food wrapped or stored in plastic), sustained stress, cigarettes and air pollution, and not eating enough fresh vegetables and fruit, which contain

antioxidants (because the body uses the antioxidants to neutralise the toxins in our body).
8. Finnerup, N. B., Attal, N., Haroutounian, S., McNicol, E., Baron, R., Dworkin, R. H., Wallace, M. (2015). Pharmacotherapy for neuropathic pain in adults: a systematic review and meta-analysis. *The Lancet. Neurology, 14*(2), 162–173.
9. Derry, S., Cording, M., Wiffen, P.J., Law, S., Phillips, T., Moore, R., (2016) Pregabalin for treating fibromyalgia pain in adults. *Cochrane*, Sept 2016.

2. Stressed out

1. Martínez, E., Aira, Z., Buesa, I., Aizpurua, I., Rada, D., & Azkue, J. J. (2018). Embodied pain in fibromyalgia: Disturbed somatorepresentations and increased plasticity of the body schema. *PloS one, 13*(4), e0194534.
2. Qin, Y., Karst, H. and Joëls, M. (2004), Chronic unpredictable stress alters gene expression in rat single dentate granule cells. Journal of Neurochemistry, 89: 364-374.
3. Schreier, H. M., & Wright, R. J. (2014). Stress and food allergy: mechanistic considerations. *Annals of allergy, asthma & immunology: Official publication of the American College of Allergy, Asthma, & Immunology, 112*(4), 296–301.
4. Mawdsley, J. E., Macey, M. G., Feakins, R.M., Langmead, L. & Rampton, D.S. (2006) The Effect of Acute Psychologic Stress on Systemic and Rectal Mucosal Measures of Inflammation in Ulcerative Colitis. *Gastroenterology.* Volume 131, Issue 2, 410 - 419
5. Thayer J.F., Lane R.D. (2007) The role of vagal function in the risk for cardiovascular disease and mortality. *Biological Psychology,* 2007 Feb;74(2):224-42. Epub 2006 Dec 19.
6. Thayer, J.F, Ahs, F, Fredrikson, M, Sollers, J.J 3rd & Wager, T.D. (2012) A meta-analysis of heart rate variability and neuroimaging studies: Implications for heart rate variability as a marker of stress and health. *Neuroscience and Biobehavioural Reviews.* 2012 Feb;36(2):747-56. Epub 2011 Dec 8.
7. Ruiz-Padial, E., Sollers J.J 3rd, Vila, J., Thayer, J.F., (2003) The rhythm of the heart in the blink of an eye: emotion-modulated startle magnitude covaries with heart rate variability. *Psychophysiology.* Mar;40(2):306-13.
8. Tracy, L.M., Ioannou, L., Baker, K.S., Gibson, S.J., Georgiou-Karistianis, N., Giummarra, M.J. (2016) Meta-analytic evidence for decreased heart rate variability in chronic pain implicating parasympathetic nervous system dysregulation. *Clinical Journal of Pain.* 2016 Jan;157(1):7-29.
9. Staud R. (2008) Heart rate variability as a biomarker of fibromyalgia syndrome. *Future Rheumatology,* 3(5), 475–483.
10. Ernst G. (2017). Heart-Rate Variability-More than Heart Beats? *Frontiers in public health, 5,* 240.
11. Ahlman, H. & Dahlstrom, A. (1983) Vagal mechanisms controlling serotonin release from the gastrointestinal tract and pyloric motor function. *Journal of the Autonomic Nervous System,* Vol 9:1 pp.119-140

12. McCraty, R & Zayas, M. A. (2014) *Cardiac coherence, self-regulation, autonomic stability, and psychological well-being.* Frontiers in Psychology, 29 Sept 2014.
13. Mogilevski, T., Burgell, R., Aziz, O., Gibson, P.R., (2019) Review article: the role of the autonomic nervous system in the pathogenesis and therapy of IBD. *Alimentary Pharmacology and Therapeutics.* First published: 16 August 2019.
14. Koopman, F. A., Chavan, S. S., Miljko, S., Grazio, S., Sokolovic, S., Schuurman, P. R., Mehta, A.D., Levine, Y A., Faltys, M., Zitnik, R., Tracey, K.J., Tak, P. P. (2016). Vagus nerve stimulation inhibits cytokine production and attenuates disease severity in rheumatoid arthritis. *Proceedings of the National Academy of Sciences of the United States of America, 113*(29), 8284–8289.
15. Oshinsky, M. L., Murphy, A. L., Hekierski, H., Jr, Cooper, M., & Simon, B. J. (2014). Noninvasive vagus nerve stimulation as treatment for trigeminal allodynia. *Pain, 155*(5), 1037–1042.

3. Trauma and fibromyalgia

1. Cuijpers, P., Smit, F., Unger, F., Stikkelbroek, Y., Ten Have, M., de Graaf, R. (2011) The disease burden of childhood adversities in adults: a population-based study. *Child Abuse & Neglect.* 2011 Nov;35(11):937-45.
2. Porges, S. (2011) *The Polyvagal Theory: Neurophysiological Foundations of Emotions, Attachment, Communication, and Self-Regulation.* W.W. Norton & Co. Series on Interpersonal Neurobiology.
3. Schauer, M. & Elbert, T. (2010). Dissociation Following Traumatic Stress. *Zeitschrift für Psychologie.* 218. 10.1027/0044-3409/a000018.
4. Vögtle, E., Kröner-Herwig, B., Barke, A. (2019). Nocebo Hyperalgesia can be Induced by the Observation of a Model Showing Natural Pain Expressions. *The Clinical Journal of Pain.* Sept 2019 - Vol 35:9. pp 737–743
5. Nasca, C., Zelli, D., Bigio, B., Piccinin,S., Scaccianoce, S., Nisticò, R., McEwen, B. S. (2015) Stress reveals a window of epigenetic plasticity. *Proceedings of the National Academy of Sciences,* Dec 2015, 112 (48) 14960-14965;
6. Porges, S. W., & Kolacz, J. (2018) 'Neurocardiology through the lens of the polyvagal theory. In, Gelpi RJ, Buchholz B. Neurocardiology: Pathophysiological Aspects and Clinical Implications. *Elsevier, Spain.* ISBN: 978-84-9113-155-7 (In press, 2018).
7. Yong-Ku, K., Kyong-Sae, N. (2016) Role of glutamate receptors and glial cells in the pathophysiology of treatment-resistant depression. *Progress in Neuro-psychopharmacology & Biological Psychiatry.* 2016 Oct 3;70:117-26
8. Li, T., Chen, X., Zhang, C. *et al.* (2019) An update on reactive astrocytes in chronic pain. *Journal of Neuroinflammation* 16, 140.
9. Stowell, R. D., Sipe, G. O., Dawes, R. P., Batchelor, H. N., Lordy, K. A., Whitelaw, B. S., Stoessel, M. B., Bidlack, J. M., Brown, E., Sur, M., & Majewska, A. K. (2019). Noradrenergic signaling in the wakeful state inhibits microglial surveillance and synaptic plasticity in the mouse visual cortex. *Nature neuroscience, 22*(11), 1782–1792.

10. Abbink, M.R., Deijk, A-LF., Heine, V.M., Verheijen, M.H., Korosi, A. (2019) The involvement of astrocytes in early-life adversity induced programming of the brain. *Glia.* 2019; 67: 1637– 1653.
11. Henn, A., Kirner, S. Leist, M. (2011) TLR2 Hypersensitivity of Astrocytes as Functional Consequence of Previous Inflammatory Episodes. *The Journal of Immunology,* March 1, 2011, 186 (5) 3237-3247.
12. Loggia, M.L., Chonde, D.B., Akeju, O., Arabasz, G., Catana, C., Edwards, R.R., Hill, E., Hsu, S., Izquierdo-Garcia, D., Ji, R.R., et al. (2015) Evidence for brain glial activation in chronic pain patients. *Brain.* 138 Pt 3:604–615.

4. Structural causes

1. Brummett, C. M., Janda, A. M., Schueller, C. M., Tsodikov, A., Morris, M., Williams, D. A., & Clauw, D. J. (2013). Survey criteria for fibromyalgia independently predict increased postoperative opioid consumption after lower-extremity joint arthroplasty: a prospective, observational cohort study. *Anesthesiology, 119*(6), 1434–1443.
2. Stecco, C., Fede, C., Macchi, V., Porzionato, A., Petrelli, L., Biz, C., Stern, R. and De Caro, R. (2018), The fasciacytes: A new cell devoted to fascial gliding regulation. *Clinical Anatomy,* 31: 667-676.
3. Temple-Wong, M.M., Ren, S., Quach, P., Hansen, B.C., Chen, A. C., Hasegawa, A. D'Lima, D. D., Koziol, J., Masuda, K., Lotz, M. K., Sah, R. L., (2016) Hyaluronan concentrations and size distribution in human knee synovial fluid: Variations with age and cartilage degeneration. *Arthritis Research and Therapy* 18:18
4. Yaron I1, Buskila D, Shirazi I, Neumann L, Elkayam O, Paran D, Yaron M. (1997) Elevated levels of hyaluronic acid in the sera of women with fibromyalgia. *Journal of Rheumatology* Nov;24 (11):2221-4.
5. Langevin, H. M. and Yandow, J. A. (2002), Relationship of acupuncture points and meridians to connective tissue planes. *Anatomical Record,* 269: 257-265.
6. Yu Bai, Jun Wang, Jin-peng Wu, et al., (2011) Review of Evidence Suggesting That the Fascia Network Could Be the Anatomical Basis for Acupoints and Meridians in the Human Body. *Evidence-Based Complementary and Alternative Medicine,* vol. 2011, Article ID 260510, 6 pages, 2011.
7. Liptan GL. Fascia: A missing link in our understanding of the pathology of fibromyalgia. *Journal of Bodywork and Movement Therapy.* 2010;14(1):3-12.
8. Doan, R.A., Monk, K.R., (2019) Glia in the skin activate pain responses. *Science* 16 Aug 2019: Vol. 365, Issue 6454, pp. 641-642
9. Abdo, H., Calvo-Enrique, L., Lopez, J.M., Song, J., Zhang, M.D., Usoskin, D., El Manira, A., Adameyko, I., Hjerling-Leffler, J., Ernfors, P. (2019) Specialized cutaneous Schwann cells initiate pain sensation. *Science* 16 Aug 2019 : 695-699
10. Campana, W. M., Mantuano, E., Azmoon, P., Henry, K., Banki, M. A., Kim, J. H., … Gonias, S. L. (2017). Ionotropic glutamate receptors activate cell signaling in response to glutamate in Schwann cells. *FASEB journal : official publication of the Federation of American Societies for Experimental Biology, 31*(4), 1744–1755.

11. Kim, S.H., Kim, D.H., Oh, D.H., Clauw, D.J., (2008) Characteristic electron microscopic findings in the skin of patients with fibromyalgia--preliminary study. Clinical Rheumatology, 2008 Mar;27(3):407-11.
12. Topp, K. & Boyd, B. (2006). Structure and Biomechanics of Peripheral Nerves: Nerve Responses to Physical Stresses and Implications for Physical Therapist Practice. Physical therapy. 86. 92-109.
13. Bordoni, B & Bordoni, G. (2015) Reflections on osteopathic fascia treatment in the peripheral nervous system. *Journal of Pain Research,* 2015:8 735-740.

5. Helping our autonomic nervous system

1. Bullmore, E. (2018) The Inflamed Mind: A Radical New Approach to Depression. *Short Books.*

6. A pain that I'm used to

1. Walder, R. Y., Rasmussen, L. A., Rainier, J. D., Light, A. R., Wemmie, J. A., & Sluka, K. A. (2010). ASIC1 and ASIC3 play different roles in the development of Hyperalgesia after inflammatory muscle injury. *The Journal of Pain: Official journal of the American Pain Society, 11*(3), 210–218.
2. Sluka, K. A., & Clauw, D. J. (2016). Neurobiology of fibromyalgia and chronic widespread pain. *Neuroscience, 338,* 114–129.
3. Woolf C. J. (2011). Central sensitization: implications for the diagnosis and treatment of pain. *Pain, 152*(3 Suppl), S2–S15.
4. Roeckel, L.A., Le Coz, G.M., Gavériaux-Ruff, C., Simonin, F. (2016). Opioid-induced hyperalgesia: Cellular and molecular mechanisms. *Neuroscience.* 338. 10.1016
5. Pereira, M. P., Donahue, R. R., Dahl, J. B., Werner, M., Taylor, B. K., & Werner, M. U. (2015). Endogenous Opioid-Masked Latent Pain Sensitization: Studies from Mouse to Human. *PloS one, 10*(8), e0134441.
6. Schrepf, A., Harper, D.E., Harte, S.E., Wang, Ichesco, H.E., Hampson, J.P., Zubieta, J-K, Clauw, D. J., & Harris, R.E. (2016) Endogenous opioidergic dysregulation of pain in fibromyalgia: a PET and fMRI study. *Pain.* 2016 October ; 157(10): 2217–2225.
7. Silverman, S.M., Hansen, H., Lee, M., Patel, V.P., & Manchikanti, L. (2011) A Comprehensive Review of Opioid-Induced Hyperalgesia. *Pain Physician* 2011;14; 145-161.
8. Vachon-Presseau, E., Berger, S. E., Abdullah, T. B., Huang, L., Cecchi, G. A., Griffith, J. W., … Apkarian, A. V. (2018). Brain and psychological determinants of placebo pill response in chronic pain patients. *Nature communications, 9*(1), 3397.
9. Vachon-Presseau E, Berger SE, Abdullah TB, Griffith JW, Schnitzer TJ, et al. (2019) Identification of traits and functional connectivity-based neurotraits of chronic pain. PLOS Biology 17(8)

10. Ossipov, M. H. (2012) The Perception and Endogenous Modulation of Pain. *Scientifica.* Vol 2012, Article ID 561761
11. Z. Q. Zhao, "Neural mechanism underlying acupuncture analgesia," *Progress in Neurobiology*, vol. 85, no. 4, pp. 355–375, 2008.
12. Tétreault, P., Mansour, A., Vachon-Presseau, E., Schnitzer, T.J., Apkarian, A.V., et al. (2016) Brain Connectivity Predicts Placebo Response across Chronic Pain Clinical Trials. *PLOS Biology* 14(10): e1002570
13. 'Opioids Aware' online resource (2020). *The Faculty of Pain Medicine, Royal College of Anaesthetists.* https://fpm.ac.uk/opioids-aware.

7. Everybody hurts

1. Lorimer, M., & Vlaeyen, J.W., (2015). Beyond nociception: the imprecision hypothesis chronic pain. *Journal of Pain.* 156. 10.1016
2. Madden, V.J., Harvie, D.S., Parker, R., Jensen, K.B., Vlaeyen, J.W.S., Moseley, G.L., Stanton, T.R., (2016) Can Pain or Hyperalgesia Be a Classically Conditioned Response in Humans? A Systematic Review and Meta-Analysis, *Pain Medicine*, Volume 17, Issue 6, June 2016, Pages 1094-1111.
3. Brinjikji, W., Luetmer, P. H., Comstock, B., Bresnahan, B. W., Chen, L. E., Deyo, R. A., Jarvik, J. G. (2015). Systematic literature review of imaging features of spinal degeneration in asymptomatic populations. *AJNR. American journal of neuroradiology*, *36*(4), 811–816.
4. Jensen, K., Kirsch, I., Odmalm, S., Kaptchuk, T. J., & Ingvar, M. (2015). Classical conditioning of analgesic and hyperalgesic pain responses without conscious awareness. *Proceedings of the National Academy of Sciences of the United States of America*, *112*(25).
5. Madden, V.J., Harvie, D.S., Parker, R., Jensen, K.B., Vlaeyen, J.W.S., Moseley, G.L., Stanton, T.R., (2016) Can Pain or Hyperalgesia Be a Classically Conditioned Response in Humans? A Systematic Review and Meta-Analysis, *Pain Medicine*, Volume 17, Issue 6, June 2016, Pages 1094-1111.

8. Illusions and interoception

1. Fang, W., Zhang, R., Zhao, Y., Wang, L., & Zhou, Y. D. (2019). Attenuation of Pain Perception Induced by the Rubber Hand Illusion. *Frontiers in neuroscience*, *13*, 261.
2. Martínez, E., Aira, Z., Buesa, I., Aizpurua, I., Rada, D., & Azkue, J. J. (2018). Embodied pain in fibromyalgia: Disturbed somatorepresentations and increased plasticity of the body schema. *PloS one*, *13*(4), e0194534.
3. Cowie D., Sterling S., Bremner A. J. The development of multisensory body representation and awareness continues to 10years of age: Evidence from the rubber hand illusion. *Journal of Experimental Child Psychology*. 2016;142:230–238.

4. Metral, M., Gonthier, C., Luyat, M., & Guerraz, M. (2017). Body Schema Illusions: A Study of the Link between the Rubber Hand and Kinesthetic Mirror Illusions through Individual Differences. *BioMed research international, 2017*, 6937328.
5. Schann, V., Schulz, A., Rubel, J. A., Bernstein, M.J., Domes, G., Schachinger, H., & Vogele, C. (2019) Childhood trauma affects stress-related interoception. *Frontiers in Psychiatry.* Received: 19 May 2019; Accepted: 18 Sep 2019.
6. Saariaho, T. H., Saariaho, A. S., Karila, I. A. and Joukamaa, M. I. (2011), Early maladaptive schemas in Finnish adult chronic pain patients and a control sample. *Scandinavian Journal of Psychology,* 52: 146-153.
7. Driskell, J., Copper, C & Moran, A. (1994). Does Mental Practice Enhance Performance? *Journal of Applied Psychology.* 79. 481-492.
8. Schwoebel, J., Friedman, R., Duda, N.H., Coslett, B. (2001) Pain and the body schema: Evidence for peripheral effects on mental representations of movement, *Brain,* Volume 124, Issue 10, October 2001, Pages 2098–2104.

9. Recap

1. Borsook, D., Youssef, A. M., Barakat, N., Sieberg, C. B., & Elman, I. (2018). Subliminal (latent) processing of pain and its evolution to conscious awareness. *Neuroscience and biobehavioral reviews, 88*, 1–15.
2. Craig, A.D. (2015) How Do You Feel? An interoceptive moment with your neurobiological self. *Princetown University Press.*
3. Thayer JF1, Ahs F, Fredrikson M, Sollers JJ 3rd, Wager TD. (2012) A meta-analysis of heart rate variability and neuroimaging studies: implications for heart rate variability as a marker of stress and health. *Neuroscience Biobehaviour Review.* 2012 Feb;36(2):747-56.

10. Inflammation and fibromyalgia

1. Bennett, J. M., Reeves, G., Billman, G. E., & Sturmberg, J. P. (2018). Inflammation-Nature's Way to Efficiently Respond to All Types of Challenges: Implications for Understanding and Managing "the Epidemic" of Chronic Diseases. *Frontiers in medicine, 5*, 316.
2. McEwen, B.S. (1999) Stress and hippocampal plasticity. *Annual Review of Neuroscience* 1999; 22: 105–122.
3. Haroon, E., Miller, A. H., & Sanacora, G. (2017). Inflammation, Glutamate, and Glia: A Trio of Trouble in Mood Disorders. *Neuropsychopharmacology: Official publication of the American College of Neuropsychopharmacology, 42*(1), 193–215.
4. Walker, A. K., Kavelaars, A., Heijnen, C. J., & Dantzer, R. (2013). Neuroinflammation and comorbidity of pain and depression. *Pharmacological reviews, 66*(1), 80–101.
5. Dantzer, R., & Walker, A. K. (2014). Is there a role for glutamate-mediated

excitotoxicity in inflammation-induced depression? *Journal of neural transmission (Vienna, Austria : 1996)*, *121*(8), 925–932.

6. Haroon, E., Miller, A. H., & Sanacora, G. (2017). Inflammation, Glutamate, and Glia: A Trio of Trouble in Mood Disorders. *Neuropsychopharmacology : official publication of the American College of Neuropsychopharmacology*, *42*(1), 193–215.
7. Bullmore, E. (2018) 'The Inflamed Mind'. Short Books
8. Balter *et al.* (2019) Selective effects of acute low-grade inflammation on human visual attention. *NeuroImage.* DOI: https://doi.org/10.1016/j.neuroimage.2019.116098
9. Maggio, M., Guralnik, J. M., Longo, D. L., & Ferrucci, L. (2006). Interleukin-6 in aging and chronic disease: a magnificent pathway. *The journals of gerontology. Series A, Biological sciences and medical sciences*, *61*(6).
10. Krueger J. M. (2008). The role of cytokines in sleep regulation. *Current pharmaceutical design*, *14*(32), 3408–3416.
11. Savitz, J. & Harrison, N. A. (2018) Interoception and Inflammation in Psychiatric Disorders. *Biological Psychiatry, Cognitive Neuroscience and Neuroimaging.* 2018 Jun; 3(6): 514–524.
12. Buric, I., Farias, M., Jong, J., Mee, C., & Brazil, I. A. (2017). What Is the Molecular Signature of Mind-Body Interventions? A Systematic Review of Gene Expression Changes Induced by Meditation and Related Practices. *Frontiers in immunology*, *8*, 670.
13. Armour, M., Smith, C. A., Wang, L-Q., Naidoo,. D., Yang, G-Y., MacPherson, H., Lee, M.S. & Hay, P. (2019) Acupuncture for Depression: A Systematic Review and Meta-Analysis. *Journal of Clinical Medicine.* 2019 Aug; 8(8): 1140.
14. Derry, S., Wiffen, P. J., Häuser, W., Mücke, M., Tölle, T. R., Bell, R. F., & Moore, R. A. (2017). Oral nonsteroidal anti-inflammatory drugs for fibromyalgia in adults. *The Cochrane database of systematic reviews*, *3*(3), CD012332.
15. Bäckryd, E., Tanum, L., Lind, A. L., Larsson, A., & Gordh, T. (2017). Evidence of both systemic inflammation and neuroinflammation in fibromyalgia patients, as assessed by a multiplex protein panel applied to the cerebrospinal fluid and to plasma. *Journal of pain research*, *10*, 515–525.

11. Calming inflammation

1. Vylkova, S., Carman, A.J., Danhof, H.A., Collette,J .R., Zhou, H., Michael C. Lorenz, M.C. (2011) The Fungal Pathogen *Candida albicans* Autoinduces Hyphal Morphogenesis by Raising Extracellular Ph. *mBio - American Society for Microbiology.* May 2011, 2 (3) e00055-11.
2. Kumamoto C.K. (2011) Inflammation and gastrointestinal *Candida* colonization. Current Opinion in Microbiology. 2011 Aug; 14(4): 386–391.
3. Lattanzio S. M. (2017). Fibromyalgia Syndrome: A Metabolic Approach Grounded in Biochemistry for the Remission of Symptoms. *Frontiers in medicine*, *4*, 198.
4. Aeberli, I., Gerber, P.A., Hochuli, M., Kohler, S., Haile, S. R., Gouni-Berthold, I.,

Berthold, H.K., Spinas, G.A., Berneis, K. (2011) Low to moderate sugar-sweetened beverage consumption impairs glucose and lipid metabolism and promotes inflammation in healthy young men: a randomized controlled trial, *The American Journal of Clinical Nutrition*, Volume 94, Issue 2, August 2011, Pages 479–485

5. Suez, J., Korem, T., Zeevi, D. *et al.* (2014) Artificial sweeteners induce glucose intolerance by altering the gut microbiota. *Nature* 514, 181–186 (2014)
6. Imamura, F., O'Connor, L., Ye, Z., Mursu, J., Hayashino, Y., Bhupathiraju, S. N., & Forouhi, N. G. (2015). Consumption of sugar sweetened beverages, artificially sweetened beverages, and fruit juice and incidence of type 2 diabetes: systematic review, meta-analysis, and estimation of population attributable fraction. *BMJ (Clinical research ed.), 351*, h3576.
7. https://www.universityofcalifornia.edu/news/americas-most-widely-consumed-cooking-oil-causes-genetic-changes-brain.
8. Lauretti E, Nenov M, Dincer O, Iuliano L, Praticò D. Extra virgin olive oil improves synaptic activity, short-term plasticity, memory, and neuropathology in a tauopathy model. *Aging Cell.* 2020;19(1):e13076.
9. Siriwardhana N, Kalupahana NS, Moustaid-Moussa N. Health benefits of n-3 polyunsaturated fatty acids: eicosapentaenoic acid and docosahexaenoic acid. *Adv Food Nutr Res.* 2012;65:211-222.
10. Hadjivassiliou, M., Grünewald, R.A., Davies-Jones, G.A.B (2002) Gluten sensitivity as a neurological illness. *Journal of Neurology, Neurosurgery & Psychiatry* 2002;72:560-563.
11. Hadjivassiliou M., Grünewald R.A., Davies-Jones G.A.B. (2002) Gluten sensitivity as a neurological illness. *Journal of Neurology, Neurosurgery & Psychiatry* 2002;72:560-563.
12. Isasi, C., Colmenero, I., Casco, F., Tejerina, E., Fernandez, N., Serrano-Vela, J. I., Villa, L. F. (2014) Fibromyalgia and non-celiac gluten sensitivity: a description with remission of fibromyalgia. *Rheumatology international, 34*(11).
13. Malekinejad H, Rezabakhsh A. Hormones in Dairy Foods and Their Impact on Public Health - A Narrative Review Article. *Iran J Public Health.* 2015;44(6):742-758.

12. Other causes of inflammation

1. Bokarewa, M. I., Erlandsson, M. C., Bjersing, J., Dehlin, M., & Mannerkorpi, K. (2014). Smoking is associated with reduced leptin and neuropeptide Y levels and higher pain experience in patients with fibromyalgia. *Mediators of inflammation, 2014*, 627041.
2. Stejskal, Vera & Ockert, Karin & Bjorklund, Geir (2013) Metal-induced inflammation triggers fibromyalgia in metal-allergic patients. *Neuro endocrinology letters.* 34. 559-65.
3. Sidoryk-Wegrzynowicz, M., & Aschner, M. (2013). Manganese toxicity in the central nervous system: the glutamine/glutamate-γ-aminobutyric acid cycle. *Journal of internal medicine*, 273(5), 466–477.

4. Kazuki, H., Taichi, K., Takashi, T. (2016) Gliotransmitter release from astrocytes: functional, developmental and pathological implications in the brain. *Frontiers in Neuroscience* Vol:9:499
5. Singh, M., & Su, C. (2013). Progesterone and neuroprotection. *Hormones and behavior, 63*(2), 284–290.
6. Schumacher, M., Hussain, R., Gago, N., Oudinet, J. P., Mattern, C., & Ghoumari, A. M. (2012). Progesterone synthesis in the nervous system: implications for myelination and myelin repair. *Frontiers in neuroscience, 6*, 10.
7. Peltier, M. R., & Sofuoglu, M. (2018). Role of Exogenous Progesterone in the Treatment of Men and Women with Substance Use Disorders: A Narrative Review. *CNS drugs, 32*(5), 421–435.
8. Perego, C., Di Cairano, E.S., Ballabio, M., Magnaghi, V. (2012) Neurosteroid allopregnanolone regulates EAAC1-mediated glutamate uptake and triggers actin changes in Schwann cells. *Journal of Cell Physiology.* 2012 Apr;227(4):1740-51.
9. Schertzinger, M., Wesson-Sides, K., Parkitny, L., & Younger, J. (2018). Daily Fluctuations of Progesterone and Testosterone Are Associated With Fibromyalgia Pain Severity. *The journal of pain : official journal of the American Pain Society, 19*(4), 410–417.
10. Ref: Okifuji, A., Turk, D.C. (2006) Sex hormones and pain in regularly menstruating women with fibromyalgia syndrome. *Journal of Pain.* 2006;7(11):851-859.
11. Gravanis, A. G. & Mellon, S. H. (2011) Hormones in Neurodegeneration, Neuroprotection, and Neurogenesis. Wiley.
12. Pluchino N, Luisi M, Lenzi E, Centofanti M, Begliuomini S, Freschi L, Ninni F, Genazzani AR.(2006) Progesterone and progestins: effects on brain, allopregnanolone and beta-endorphin. *Journal of Steroid Biochemistry Molecular Biology* 2006 Dec;102(1-5):205-13. Epub 2006 Oct 18.
13. Pluchino N, Luisi M, Lenzi E, Centofanti M, Begliuomini S, Freschi L, Ninni F, Genazzani AR.(2006) Progesterone and progestins: effects on brain, allopregnanolone and beta-endorphin. *Journal of Steroid Biochemistry Molecular Biology* 2006 Dec;102(1-5):205-13. Epub 2006 Oct 18.
14. Porcu, P., Mostallino, M.C., Sogliano, C., Santoru, F., Berretti, R., Concas, A. (2012) Long-term administration with levonorgestrel decreases allopregnanolone levels and alters GABAA receptor subunit expression and anxiety-like behavior. *Pharmacology Biochemistry and Behaviour,* Vol 102:2, p 366-372.
15. Pinna, G., & Rasmusson, A. M. (2012). Up-regulation of neurosteroid biosynthesis as a pharmacological strategy to improve behavioural deficits in a putative mouse model of post-traumatic stress disorder. *Journal of neuroendocrinology, 24*(1), 102–116.
16. Naylor, J.C., Kilts, J.D., Szabo, S.T., Dunn, C.E., Keefe, F.J., Tupler, L.A., Shampine, L.J., Morey, R.A., Strauss, J.L., Hamer, R.M., Wagner, H.R., MIRECC Workgroup, Marx, C.E., (2016) Allopregnanolone Levels Are Inversely Associated with Self-Reported Pain Symptoms in U.S. Iraq and Afghanistan-Era Veterans: Implications for Biomarkers and Therapeutics, *Pain Medicine*, Volume 17, Issue 1, January 2016, Pages 25–32.

17. Giatti, S., Melcangi, R.C., & Pesaresi, M. (2016) The other side of progestins: effects in the brain. *Journal of Molecular Endocrinology*, Vol 57:2
18. Perlmutter, D., Loberg, K. (2014) Grain Brain. Yellow Kite.
19. Dong, E., Matsumoto, K., Uzunova, V., Sugaya, I., Takahata, H., Nomura, H., Guidotti, A. (2001). Brain 5alpha-dihydroprogesterone and allopregnanolone synthesis in a mouse model of protracted social isolation. *Proceedings of the National Academy of Sciences of the United States of America, 98*(5), 2849–2854.
20. Rasmusson, A. M., Pinna, G., Paliwal, P., Weisman, D., Gottschalk, C., Charney, D., Krystal, J., Guidotti A. (2006) Decreased Cerebrospinal Fluid Allopregnanolone Levels in Women with Posttraumatic Stress Disorder. *Biological Psychiatry*, Volume 60, Issue 7, 704 - 713
21. Naylor, J.C., Kilts, J.D., Szabo, S.T., Dunn, C.E., Keefe, F.J., Tupler, L.A., Shampine, L.J., Morey, R.A., Strauss, J.L., Hamer, R.M., Wagner, H.R., MIRECC Workgroup, Marx, C.E., (2016) Allopregnanolone Levels Are Inversely Associated with Self-Reported Pain Symptoms in U.S. Iraq and Afghanistan-Era Veterans: Implications for Biomarkers and Therapeutics, *Pain Medicine*, Volume 17, Issue 1, January 2016, Pages 25–32.
22. Brown S.L., Fredrickson B.L., Wirth M.M., Poulin M.J., Meier E.A., Heaphy E.D., Cohen M.D., Schultheiss O.C. (2009) Social closeness increases salivary progesterone in humans. *Hormonal Behaviour.* 2009;56:108–111.
23. *Zak P.J., Kurzban. R., Matzner. W.T. (2005)* Oxytocin is associated with human trustworthiness.
Hormonal Behaviour. 2005 Dec; 48(5):522-7.
24. Berta, T., Qadri, Y. J., Chen, G., & Ji, R. R. (2016). Microglial Signaling in Chronic Pain with a Special Focus on Caspase 6, p38 MAP Kinase, and Sex Dependence. *Journal of dental research, 95*(10), 1124–1131.
25. Matteson, E. L., et al. (2012) Patient-reported Outcomes in Polymyalgia Rheumatica. *The Journal of Rheumatology* Apr 2012, 39 (4) 795-803.
26. Marsman, D.E., den Broeder, N., Boers, N., van den Hoogen, F.H.J, den Broeder, A.A., van der Maas, A. (2020) Polymyalgia rheumatica patients with and without elevated baseline acute phase reactants: distinct subgroups of polymyalgia rheumatica? Clinical & Experimental Rheumatology, 2020 Apr 3.
27. Xia, S., Zhang, X., Zheng, S., Khanabdali, R., Kalionis, B., Wu, J., Wan, W., & Tai, X. (2016). An Update on Inflamm-Aging: Mechanisms, Prevention, and Treatment. *Journal of immunology research, 2016*, 8426874.
28. Coskun Benlidayi, I. Role of inflammation in the pathogenesis and treatment of fibromyalgia. *Rheumatology International* 39, 781–791 (2019).
29. Brebner, K., Hayley, S., Zacharko, R. *et al.* Synergistic Effects of Interleukin-1β, Interleukin-6, and Tumor Necrosis Factor-α: Central Monoamine, Corticosterone, and Behavioral Variations. *Neuropsychopharmacology* 22, 566–580 (2000).
30. Hutchings, A., Hollywood, J., Lamping, D.L., Pease, C.T., Chakravarty, K., Silverman, B., Choy, E.H.S., Scott, D.G.I., Hazleman, B.L., Bourke, B., Gendi, N. and Dasgupta, B. (2007), Clinical outcomes, quality of life, and diagnostic uncertainty in the first year of polymyalgia rheumatica. *Arthritis & Rheumatism,* 57: 803-809.
31. Häuser, W., Perrot, S., Sommer, C., Shir, Y., & Fitzcharles, M. A. (2017).

Diagnostic confounders of chronic widespread pain: not always fibromyalgia. *Pain reports, 2*(3), e598.

13. Reboot your brain

1. Davis M. (2011). NMDA receptors and fear extinction: implications for cognitive behavioral therapy. *Dialogues in clinical neuroscience, 13*(4), 463–474.
2. van den Broeke, E.N., Geene, N.,van Rijn, C.M., Wilder-Smith, O.H., Oosterman, J. (2014) Negative expectations facilitate mechanical hyperalgesia after high-frequency electrical stimulation of human skin. *European Journal of Pain.* 2014 Jan;18(1):86-91.
3. Bąbel, P., Adamczyk, W., Świder, K., Bajcar, E.A., Kicman, P., Lisińska, N., (2018) How Classical Conditioning Shapes Placebo Analgesia: Hidden versus Open Conditioning, *Pain Medicine*, Volume 19, Issue 6, June 2018, Pages 1156–1169, https://doi.org/10.1093/pm/pnx177
4. Myers, K. M., Carlezon, W. A., Jr, & Davis, M. (2011). Glutamate receptors in extinction and extinction-based therapies for psychiatric illness. *Neuropsychopharmacology : official publication of the American College of Neuropsychopharmacology, 36*(1), 274–293. doi:10.1038/npp.2010.88
5. van de Kolk, B, (2015) The Body keeps the Score; Mind, Brain and Body in the transformation of Trauma. *Penguin.* p.121.
6. Schauer, M. & Elbert, T. (2010). Dissociation Following Traumatic Stress. *Zeitschrift für Psychologie.* 218. 10.1027/0044-3409/a000018.
7. 58 Serra J, Bostock H, Sola R, Aleu J, Garcia E, Cokic B, Navarro X, Quiles C. (2012) Microneurographic identification of spontaneous activity in C-nociceptors in neuropathic pain states in humans and rats. *Pain.* 2012;153:42–55.
8. Harte, S. E., Clauw, D. J., Hayes, J. M., Feldman, E. L., St Charles, I. C., & Watson, C. J. (2017). Reduced intraepidermal nerve fiber density after a sustained increase in insular glutamate: a proof-of-concept study examining the pathogenesis of small fiber pathology in fibromyalgia. *Pain reports, 2*(3), e590.
9. Häuser, W., & Fitzcharles, M. A. (2018). Facts and myths pertaining to fibromyalgia. *Dialogues in clinical neuroscience, 20*(1), 53–62.

14. What can I do now to get better?

1. Felger J. C. (2018). Imaging the Role of Inflammation in Mood and Anxiety-related Disorders. Current neuropharmacology, 16(5), 533–558
2. Bower, J. E., & Irwin, M. R. (2016). Mind-body therapies and control of inflammatory biology: A descriptive review. Brain, behavior, and immunity, 51, 1–11.
3. Chung, J.W.Y., Yan, V.C.M., & Zhang, H. (2014) Effect of Acupuncture on Heart Rate Variability: A Systematic Review. *Evidence-Based Complementary and Alternative Medicine,* Vol 2014, Article ID 819871.

4. Chambers AS, Allen JJB. (2002) Vagal tone as an indicator of treatment response in major depression. *Psychophysiology.* 2002;39:861–864.
5. Ji-Hung Wang, Terry B. J. Kuo, Cheryl C. H. Yang (2002) An alternative method to enhance vagal activities and suppress sympathetic activities in humans. *Autonomic Neuroscience,* 2002
   DOI:10.1016/S1566-0702(02)00150-9
6. Harris, R. E., Sundgren, P. C., Pang, Y., Hsu, M. , Petrou, M. , Kim, S. , McLean, S. A., Gracely, R. H. and Clauw, D. J. (2008), Dynamic levels of glutamate within the insula are associated with improvements in multiple pain domains in fibromyalgia. Arthritis & Rheumatism, 58: 903-907.
7. De Silva, M. A. H. & Dorsher, P. T. (2013) Neuroanatomic and Clinical Correspondences: Acupuncture and Vagus Nerve Stimulation. *The Journal of Alternative and Complementary Medicine.* Vol.0:0 pp.1-8.
8. Lim, H. D., Kim, M. H., Lee, C. Y., & Namgung, U. (2016). Anti-Inflammatory Effects of Acupuncture Stimulation via the Vagus Nerve. *PloS one, 11*(3), e0151882. doi:10.1371/journal.pone.0151882
9. da Silva, M. D., Bobinski, F., Sato, K. L., Kolker, S. J., Sluka, K. A., & Santos, A. R. (2015). IL-10 cytokine released from M2 macrophages is crucial for analgesic and anti-inflammatory effects of acupuncture in a model of inflammatory muscle pain. *Molecular neurobiology, 51*(1), 19–31.
10. Andersson, U., & Tracey, K. J. (2012). Neural reflexes in inflammation and immunity. *The Journal of experimental medicine, 209*(6), 1057–1068.
11. Young, H. A., & Benton, D. (2018). Heart-rate variability: a biomarker to study the influence of nutrition on physiological and psychological health? *Behavioural pharmacology, 29*(2 and 3-Spec Issue), 140–151.
12. Chu, I.H, Wu, W.L, Lin, I.M, Chang, Y.K, Lin, Y.J, Yang, P.C. (2017) Effects of Yoga on Heart Rate Variability and Depressive Symptoms in Women: A Randomized Controlled Trial. *Journal of Alternative Complementary Medicine.* 2017 Apr;23(4):310-316. doi: 10.1089/acm.2016.0135. Epub 2017 Jan 4.
13. Tyagi, A. & Cohen, M. (2016) Yoga and heart rate variability: A comprehensive review of the literature. *International Journal of Yoga.* 2016 Jul-Dec; 9(2): 97–113.
14. Deschodt-Arsac, V., Lalanne, R., Spiluttini, B., Bertin, C., & Arsac, L. M. (2018). Effects of heart rate variability biofeedback training in athletes exposed to stress of university examinations. *PloS one, 13*(7), e0201388. doi:10.1371/journal.pone.0201388
15. Dana, D, (2018) *The Polyvagal Theory in Therapy; Engaging the Rhythm of Regulation.* Norton, New York. p.97.
16. Kanbara, K., & Fukunaga, M.(2016). Links among emotional awareness, somatic awareness and autonomic homeostatic processing. *BioPsychoSocial Medicine,* 10, 16. doi:10.1186/s13030-016-0059-3
17. van de Kolk, B, (2015) The Body keeps the Score; Mind, Brain and Body in the transformation of Trauma. Penguin.
18. Barrientos, R.M., Frank, M.G., Crysdale, N.Y., Chapman, T.R., Ahrendsen, J.T., Day, H.E., Campeau, S., Watkins, L.R., Patterson, S.L., Maier, S.F. (2011) Little

exercise, big effects: reversing aging and infection-induced memory deficits, and underlying processes. *Journal of Neuroscience 31*: 11578–11586, 2011.
19. The Foundation for Peripheral Neuropathy, website: https://www.foundationforpn.org/
20. Häuser, W., & Fitzcharles, M. A. (2018). Facts and myths pertaining to fibromyalgia. *Dialogues in clinical neuroscience, 20*(1), 53–62.
21. Okan, S., Caglıyan Turk, A., Sıvgın, H., Ozsoy, F., & Okan, F. (2019). Association of ferritin levels with depression, anxiety, sleep quality, and physical functioning in patients with fibromyalgia syndrome: a cross-sectional study. *Croatian medical journal, 60*(6), 515–520.
22. *Ortancil, O., Sanli, A., Eryuksel, R. *et al.* Association between serum ferritin level and fibromyalgia syndrome. *European Journal of Clinical Nutrition* 64, 308–312 (2010).
23. Yanoff, L., Menzie, C., Denkinger, B. *et al.* Inflammation and iron deficiency in the hypoferremia of obesity. *International Journal of Obesity* 31, 1412–1419 (2007).
24. *Al-Jafar H. A. (2017). HWA: Hypoferritinemia without anemia a hidden hematology disorder. *Journal of family medicine and primary care, 6*(1), 69–72.
25. Soppi, E. T. (2018) Iron deficiency without anemia - a clinical challenge. *Clinical Case Reports* 2018; 6(6): 1082-1086
26. Oaklander, A. L., & Klein, M.M., (2013) Evidence of Small-Fiber Polyneuropathy in Unexplained, Juvenile-Onset, Widespread Pain Syndromes. *Pediatrics* Apr 2013, 131 (4) e1091-e1100; DOI: 10.1542/peds.2012-2597
27. Goldenberg D.L., Clauw D.J., Palmer R.E., Clair A.G. (2016) Opioid Use in Fibromyalgia: A Cautionary Tale. *Mayo Clinic Proceedings* 2016 May;91(5):640-8. doi: 10.1016/j.mayocp.2016.02.002. Epub 2016 Mar 11.
28. Fitzcharles, M.A., Faregh, N., Ste-Marie, P.A., & Shir, Y. "Opioid Use in Fibromyalgia Is Associated with Negative Health Related Measures in a Prospective Cohort Study," *Pain Research and Treatment,* vol. 2013, Article ID 898493, 7 pages.

15. Taking control of fibromyalgia

1. [The] "*dorsal motor nucleus of the vagus (DMV), synaptic contacts are not static but undergo plastic changes to ensure that vagally regulated gastrointestinal functions respond appropriately to ever-changing physiological conditions or derangements*" quote from; Travagli, R. A., & Anselmi, L. (2016). Vagal neurocircuitry and its influence on gastric motility. *Nature reviews. Gastroenterology & hepatology, 13*(7), 389–401. doi:10.1038/nrgastro.2016.76
2. Lyon, P., Cohen, M., Quintner, J. (2011) An Evolutionary Stress-Response Hypothesis for Chronic Widespread Pain (Fibromyalgia Syndrome), *Pain Medicine*, Vol:12: Issue 8, August 2011, Pages 1167–1178.
3. Berger, (1999) J.Herbal Rituals: Recipes for Everyday Living. St. Martin's Griffin
4. Qi, Q., Liu, Y. N., Jin, X. M., Zhang, L. S., Wang, C., Bao, C. H., Liu, H. R., Wu, H. G., & Wang, X. M. (2018). Moxibustion treatment modulates the gut

microbiota and immune function in a dextran sulphate sodium-induced colitis rat model. World journal of gastroenterology, 24(28), 3130–3144.
5. From the blog, 'The Victorian Cyclist' by William Manners, author of (2019) Revolution: How the Bicycle Reinvented Modern Britain. Duckworth.

Acupressure tools

1. Harris RE1, Tian X, Williams DA, Tian TX, Cupps TR, Petzke F, Groner KH, Biswas P, Gracely RH, Clauw DJ. (2005) Treatment of fibromyalgia with formula acupuncture: investigation of needle placement, needle stimulation, and treatment frequency. *Journal of Alternative and Complementary Medicine,* New York. Aug;11(4):663-71. [Points used: Du.20, LI.11, LI.4, GB.34, St.36, Sp.6, Liv.3]

   & Mist, S.D., Dupree Jones, K. (2018) Randomized Controlled Trial of Acupuncture for Women with Fibromyalgia: Group Acupuncture with Traditional Chinese Medicine Diagnosis-Based Point Selection. *Pain Medicine,* Volume 19, Issue 9, September 2018, Pages 1862–1871
2. Montakab, H. (2014) *Acupuncture Point and Channel Energetics, Bridging the Gap.* Kiener.
3. Keown, D. (2014) *The Spark in the Machine: How the Science of Acupuncture Explains the Mysteries of Western Medicine.* Singing Dragon. pp.274-277.
4. Xia, B., Xie, Y.,Hu, S., Xu, T., Tong, P. (2018) Effect of Auricular Point Acupressure on Axial Neck Pain After Anterior Cervical Discectomy and Fusion: A Randomized Controlled Trial, *Pain Medicine*, Volume 19, Issue 1, January 2018, Pages 193–201

MEDICAL DISCLAIMER

This book provides general information. It is not intended to be a substitute for professional medical advice and should not be relied on as personal advice. Always seek the guidance of your doctor or other qualified health professional with any questions you may have regarding your health or a medical condition. Never disregard the advice of a medical professional, or delay in seeking it because of something you have read in this book.

The information in this book is provided without any representations or warranties, express or implied. If you choose to rely on any information provided in this book, you do so solely at your own risk.

Under no circumstances is the author responsible for the claims of third party websites, books, or educational providers mentioned in this book.

Printed in Great Britain
by Amazon

48914387R00175